FRONTIERS IN REPRODUCTIVE ENDOCRINOLOGY AND INFERTILITY

T0321160

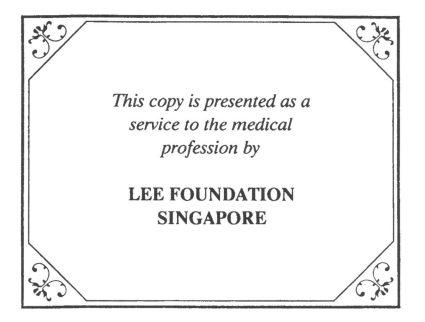

DEDICATION

This book is dedicated to our wives and families
for their support and encouragement.

FRONTIERS IN REPRODUCTIVE ENDOCRINOLOGY AND INFERTILITY

EDITORS

Charles S A Ng
MA, MBB Chir(Camb), FRCOG, AM
Senior Consultant and Head
Dept of Obstetrics and Gynecology
Singapore General Hospital
Singapore

F M Maurine Tsakok
MRCS LRCP, MBBS(Lond),
MMed (O&G), FRCOG, PhD, AM
Senior Consultant and
Deputy Head
Dept of Obstetrics and Gynecology
Singapore General Hospital
Singapore

Seang-Lin Tan
MBBS, MRCOG(Lond),
MMed (O&G), AM
Obstetrician and Gynecologist
Dept of Obstetrics and Gynecology
'B' Unit
Kandang Kerbau Hospital
Singapore

Kong-Hon Chan
MBBS, MRCOG(Lond),
MMed (O&G)
Obstetrician and
Gynecologist
Dept of Obstetrics and Gynecology
Singapore General Hospital
Singapore

KLUWER ACADEMIC PUBLISHERS

DORDRECHT - BOSTON - LONDON

Distributors

for the United States and Canada: Kluwer Academic Publishers, PO Box 358, Accord Station, Hingham, MA 02018-0358, USA
for all other countries: Kluwer Academic Publishers Group, Distribution Center, PO Box 322, 3300 AH Dordrecht, The Netherlands

ISBN 0-7462-0092-7

Copyright

Published in the United Kingdom by Kluwer Academic Publishers, PO Box 55, Lancaster, UK.

Kluwer Academic Publishers BV incorporates the publishing programmes of D. Reidel, Martinus Nijhoff, Dr W. Junk and MTP Press.

Printed and bound in Great Britain by Butler and Tanner, Frome and London

Contents

List of Contributors

David F Archer, MD
Director, Clinical Research
Contraceptive Research &
    Development Program
Dept of Obstetrics & Gynaecology
Eastern Virginia Medical School
700 Olney Road
Norfolk, Virginia 23507
USA

Marc Bygdeman, MD
Professor, Chairman
Department of Obstetrics &
    Gynaecology
Karolinska Hospital
S-10401 Stockholm
Sweden

Kong-Hon Chan, MRCOG
Obstetrician & Gynaecologist
Department of Obstetrics &
    Gynaecology
Singapore General Hospital
Singapore 0316

Ian D Cooke, FRCOG
Professor
University Department of Obstetrics
    & Gynaecology
Jessop Hospital for Women
Sheffield S3 7RE
UK

James F Daniell, MD, FACOG
Women's Health Group
2222 State Street
Nashville, Tennessee
USA

Wilfried Feichtinger, MD
Facharzt fur Frauenheilkunde und
    Geburtshilfe
Trauttmansdorffgasse 3A
A-1130 Vienna
Austria

Roger D Kempers, MD, FACOG
Professor
Department of Obstetrics &
    Gynaecology
Mayo Medical School & Mayo Clinic
Rochester, Minnesota 55905
USA;
Editor in Chief, *Fertility & Sterility*,
President Elect, American Fertility
    Society

William R Keye Jr, MD
Associate Professor
The University of Utah
Department of Obstetrics &
    Gynaecology
Room 2B200
50 North Medical Drive
Salt Lake City, Utah 84132
USA

Charles S A Ng, FRCOG
Head, Consultant Obstetrician &
   Gynaecologist
Department of Obstetrics &
   Gynaecology
Singapore General Hospital
Singapore 0316

Roger J Pepperell, MD, BS, MGO,
   MD(Mon), FRACP, FRCOG,
   FRACOG
Dept of Obstetrics & Gynaecology
University of Melbourne
Parkville, Victoria 3052
Australia

Eric J Thomas, MBBS, MRCOG
Consultant/Senior Lecturer
Newcastle General Hospital
Westgate Road
Newcastle Upon Tyne NE4 6BE
UK

F H Maurine Tsakok, PhD, FRCOG
Deputy Head, Consultant
   Obstetrician & Gynaecologist
Department of Obstetrics &
   Gynaecology
Singapore General Hospital
Singapore 0316

Preface

This book presenting the latest thinking on Reproductive Endocrinology and Infertility is truly international as the authors hail from no less than four different continents (North America, Europe, Australia and Asia).

The idea for this book was conceived during the XII World Congress On Fertility and Sterility where the unique confluence of our distinguished authors occurred in Singapore in October 1986. The authors were involved in the Pre And Post Congress Scientific Programmes which we organised.

The overwhelming success of the Congress and the Pre And Post Congress Scientific Programmes prompted this book so that those unable to attend the meeting will still be able to benefit from the vast range of topics covered.

This book will be a valuable addition to the knowledge in Reproductive Endocrinology and Infertility and will be useful reading for those wishing to pursue this subspecialty.

The authors are indebted to Lee Foundation (Singapore) for help in the publication of this book. We would also like to thank Miss Jam Siew Fong and Miss Tang May Mey for their excellent secretarial assistance.

Singapore, January 1988

                        Charles S A Ng
                        F H Maurine Tsakok
                        S L Tan
                        K H Chan

1

Hypothalamic and Pituitary Disorders in Reproduction

ROGER J PEPPERELL

Disorders of ovulation are present in 15 to 25% of couples with infertility. The vast majority of these disorders have their origin in the hypothalamus or pituitary. In many of these women, the disorder of ovulation is obvious as there is a complete lack of menstruation (primary or secondary amenorrhea); however, in others menstruation may be occurring irregularly (oligomenorrhea with cycles every 6 weeks to 6 months) or even regularly every 28 days, yet a disorder of ovulation is present. As women with cycles of longer than 6 weeks have a reduced number of ovulations per year (if they are ovulating at all), they are usually investigated and treated along the same lines as those with a complete lack of periods.

PATIENT ASSESSMENT

The basic evaluation of such women should include a skull x-ray and measurement of serum follicle-stimulating hormone (FSH), luteinizing hormone (LH), prolactin (PRL), thyroxine (T_4), tri-iodothyronine resin uptake (T_3RU) and thyroid-stimulating hormone (TSH) levels (Figure 1). The results of these investigations will usually enable the clinician to clearly define the cause of the anovulation and which treatment, if any, is indicated.

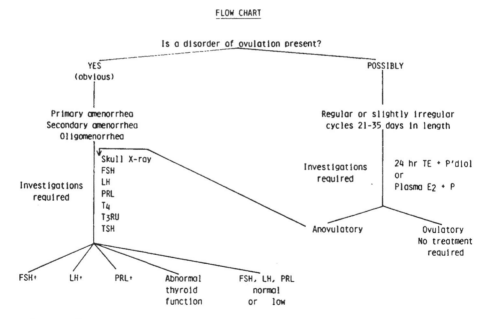

Figure 1 Evaluation of the patient with an apparent disorder of ovulation.

2

Where regular menstrual cycles are present, it is important to assess if ovulation is occurring, as approximately 5 to 10% of such women are anovulatory when assessed appropriately. This assessment should include the measurement of plasma progesterone or urinary pregnanediol in the mid-luteal phase of the cycle, values of greater than 10ng/ml and 2mg/24 hours respectively being indicative of ovulation. Provided the plasma or urine specimen is collected 4 to 10 days before the onset of the period, the values are an accurate reflection of the presence or absence of ovulation.

Where the adequacy of corpus luteum function needs to be assessed however, more than 1 plasma or urine specimen is necessary and samples are usually collected at least every third day during the whole luteal phase. There is a lack of agreement in regard to both the relevance of the deficient corpus luteum in infertile patients and what is the best treatment for this alleged condition when it is diagnosed. Because of this, further discussion of this topic will not be included.

ETIOLOGY OF OVULATORY DISORDERS

The basic causes of secondary amenorrhea are shown in Figure 2 with the common causes of the ovulatory disturbances presenting as secondary amenorrhea indicated (1). With the exception of ovarian failure, which occurs in virtually all women who reach the age of 60 years but is seen in 10% of women with secondary amenorrhea under the age of 35 years, the common causes of anovulation act at the level of the hypothalamus. Obesity is associated more with oligomenorrhea than secondary amenorrhea but severe weight loss, particularly when combined with other features of anorexia nervosa, is associated with amenorrhea. Approximately 1% of women will have at least 12 months secondary amenorrhea following cessation of the oral contraceptive pill, even when their menstrual cycles prior to commencing the pill were perfectly regular, but the incidence of secondary amenorrhea is much higher when the menstrual cycles had previously been irregular or greater than 6 weeks in length. Psychological disturbances (particularly change of employment, family arguments, exams or overseas travel) are also commonly associated with ovulatory disturbances, and excessive exercise (especially long distance running or swimming) may also cause amenorrhea.

3

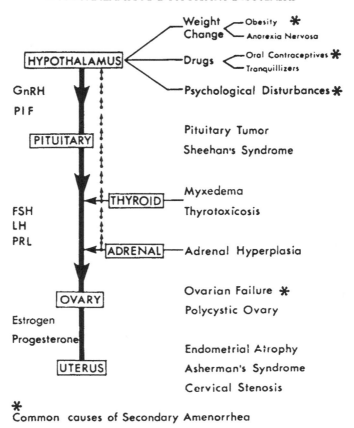

Figure 2 Etiology of secondary amenorrhea (GnRH = gonadotropin-releasing hormone; PIF = prolactin-inhibiting factor; LH = luteinizing hormone; PRL = prolactin)
*The common causes of secondary amenorrhea.

MANAGEMENT OF THE PATIENT WITH AN OVULATORY DISORDER

Investigation

As indicated above, the basic evaluation of these women should include the performance of a skull x-ray and the measurement of serum FSH, LH, PRL, T_4, T_3RU and TSH levels. Analysis of the results of the hormonal investigations allows the patients to be clearly separated into 5 distinct categories - those with elevated FSH levels, elevated LH levels, elevated PRL levels, disordered thyroid function, and those in whom FSH, LH and PRL levels are all normal or low. It is appropriate for patients to be considered in these 5 categories as each is managed in a different way.

Although a single blood sample does not provide a completely accurate value for the integrated serum FSH or LH levels over a 12- to 24-hour time interval, single samples provide valid information under most circumstances. Where the FSH level is elevated, this assay should be repeated on at least 2 more occasions before the patient is informed of the likely diagnosis. The investigation should also be repeated when the initial serum PRL level is found to be elevated - in these circumstances subsequent serum specimens should be colleted in the morning, with the patient rested both physically and emotionally. For the clinician making decisions about patient management, stimulatory tests with GnRH or thyrotropin (TRH) add little further information to that provided by the basal FSH, LH and PRL values and are thus usually unnecessary.

Where there is clinical evidence of hirsutism or virilization, serum testosterone, androstenedione and dehydroepiandrosterone sulphate (DHEAS) levels should also be measured. In the absence of hirsutism or virilization these investigations are not required.

Treatment of Patients found to have Elevated FSH Levels

When the serum FSH level is persistently elevated to values above those seen at the mid-cycle peak of the normal menstrual cycle, the diagnosis is either premature menopause or the 'resistant ovary syndrome'. The former condition is associated with a complete lack of primordial follicles in the ovaries, whereas the latter condition, the cause of which is unclear, is associated with a normal complement of primordial follicles in the ovary. Ovarian biopsy will thus usually differentiate between these conditions. However, the biopsy is best obtained as an open procedure as laparoscopic ovarian biopsy has been shown to be inaccurate if the portion of ovary obtained contains no primordial follicles when examined under the microscope. Chromosome analysis is indicated when the apparent diagnosis is premature ovarian failure as discovery of a 47 XXX or 48 XXXX chromosome complement would indicate that ovarian biopsy is not required.

Where the diagnosis of premature menopause is made, hormone replacement therapy with estrogen and progestogen may be indicated. Where the diagnosis of resistant ovary syndrome is made, however, hormone replacement therapy should be withheld, unless pregnancy is not desired, as about 64% of these patients will subsequently menstruate spontaneously and about 9% will conceive (2). There is no place for treatment with clomiphene citrate or gonadotropin as whilst the serum FSH levels are elevated, such treatment is completely ineffective. When the FSH levels fall to normal, however, spontaneous ovarian activity occurs.

Treatment of Patients found to have Elevated LH Levels

Where the LH level is elevated, consideration of the FSH level will usually allow a correct evaluation to be made. Elevation of both FSH and LH levels is usually associated with premature ovarian failure or ovarian resistance, while an elevated LH level associated with an upper normal FSH level is usually indicative of mid-cycle peaks of these hormones consistent with spontaneous cure of the anovulatory disorder. Where the LH level is markedly elevated but the FSH level is in the low normal range, an early pregnancy should be suspected as most LH assays show significant cross-reactivity between LH and human chorionic gonadotropin (hCG); where the FSH level is normal but the LH level is mildly elevated, polycystic ovarian disease is often found. The FSH and LH levels in the latter condition are also often observed in obese patients without evidence of polycystic ovarian disease and in women about to resolve their anovulatory problems spontaneously.

When ovulation induction is indicated and clomiphene citrate or gonadotrophin therapy is used, extreme care should be exercised if the LH level is moderately elevated, as hyperstimulation commonly occurs if an excessive dose of either agent is given.

Treatment of Patients found to have Elevated PRL Levels

The incidence of hyperprolactinemia in subjects with secondary amenorrhea and oligomenorrhea is 23% and 8% respectively (1). It is rarely encountered in patients with primary amenorrhea or those with regular ovulatory cycles.

Approximately 20% of amenorrheic women with elevated PRL levels can be shown to have a pituitary tumor when sophisticated radiology such as polytomography and/or computerized axial tomography (CT) scanning is used in the assessment. The accuracy of polytomography has been seriously questioned (3, 4) and CT scanning using phase 1 or phase 2 machines is of very limited value. There is now general agreement that a CT scan should be performed where the plain x-ray is abnormal or where the PRL level is elevated.

The vast majority of such pituitary tumors are small, confined within the pituitary fossa, and grow very slowly (if at all); the clinician can usually proceed to ovulation induction with bromocriptine whether a pituitary tumor is identified or not. The main risk of treatment in such patients is the possibility of a progressive increase in size of the tumor during pregnancy induced with bromocriptine therapy with resultant pressure on the optic chiasma. The risk of this is exceedingly small where the tumor is confined to the fossa prior to the pregnancy. Surgical excision or treatment of a pituitary tumor with radiotherapy is rarely necessary even when the tumor is extending out of the pituitary fossa; bromocriptine therapy usually controls tumor growth and can be continued during pregnancy if necessary. Even surgical excision does not prevent further progression of tumors in all instances (5), and many patients who apparently have complete surgical excision of microadenomas ultimately require treatment with bromocriptine because of recurrent hyperprolactinemia.

Thus, irrespective of the cause of the hyperprolactinemia (except primary hypothyroidism), bromocriptine is the treatment of choice and ovulation and pregnancy rates of 96% and 83% respectively have been reported.

Use of Bromocriptine

The drug is administered orally and the dose increased at intervals until satisfactory ovulation occurs. Apart from mild nausea and postural hypotension, the treatment is virtually free of side-effects. The incidence of multiple pregnancy is not increased and, although the drug is commonly stopped as soon as pregnancy is confirmed, no teratogenic effects have been described.

Bromocriptine is commenced in the low dose of 1.25mg (half a tablet) twice daily for one week. This is taken with meals to reduce gastrointestinal side-effects and the low dose allows the patient to become accustomed to the drug and able to tolerate higher doses. After a week, the dose is increased to 2.5mg twice daily and maintained at this level.

Approximately 4-5 weeks after commencing therapy, the response is assessed by determining the serum prolactin level, and by examining for the persistence of galactorrhea if this was present initially. If the PRL is still elevated the dose of bromocriptine is doubled to 5mg twice daily. The assessment is repeated monthly with the dose of bromocriptine being further increased progressively to a maximum of 20mg twice daily (40mg/day) where the PRL remains elevated and amenorrhea continues. Where the menses return, further assessment of PRL, and an assessment of estrogen and pregnanediol (progesterone) levels should be timed for the mid-luteal phase as an increase in dose of bromocriptine may still be necessary if the PRL level is in the upper normal range and/or the luteal phase is shown to the deficient.

Where laboratory facilities are not available, the dosage can be increased empirically until a response, as indicated by bleeding or pregnancy, is obtained. If conception does not occur within 3 to 4 months on this empirical regimen, it is necessary to reassess the situation by measurement of the serum PRL values to determine whether suppression of the hyperprolactinemia has been adequate. Most patients respond to treatment with bromocriptine at a daily dose of 5 to 10mg and the great majority who conceive do so within 6 ovulatory cycles.

Once ovulation occurs during treatment with bromocriptine regular ovulation usually continues for as long as the drug is administered or until conception results. It has been usual to stop bromocriptine as soon as a positive pregnancy test is obtained. Following cessation of this agent, serum PRL levels rise rapidly to values similar to those which were present prior to treatment and which are significantly higher than those seen at the same time in normal pregnancy. Although this elevation in prolactin levels is accompanied by a significant fall in urinary pregnanediol excretion between 11 and 14 weeks of gestation (7), all pregnancies where a fetus is present continue normally without supplemental progesterone therapy and the overall abortion rate following this treatment is not increased above normal.

The hormonal responses to therapy are illustrated in figure 3. The elevated PRL levels are rapidly suppressed to normal, and galactorrhea, if present initially, subsides. However, ovarian activity often does not commence until the serum PRL level is suppressed below 10 ng/ml. In at least half of the patients treated the initial ovarian response is not that of normal ovulation as follicular development without ovulation or ovulation with deficient corpus luteum function is observed. These partial responses may resolve into full ovulatory responses in subsequent cycles even without an increase in the dose of bromocriptine administered.

Concurrent use of other agents: Most hyperprolactinemic patients respond as illustrated above however, in about 5% of subjects, adequate PRL suppression is not associated with a return of ovarian function. Administration of clomiphene citrate, in addition to the continuing treatment with bromocriptine, commonly restores ovulation under these circumstances and it has been assumed that a dual hypothalamic-pituitary cause has been the cause of the ovulatory disorder.

In a further 5% of hyperprolactinemic subjects, the serum PRL level cannot be suppressed to normal despite the administration of exceedingly large doses of bromocriptine (up to 80mg/day). Some of these subjects have obvious suprasellar or pituitary tumors, others have small adenomas only evident with sophisticated CT scanning techniques but in many the reason for the failure of PRL suppression remains obscure. In some of these subjects the PRL level prior to treatment is only 2-3 times the upper limit of normal

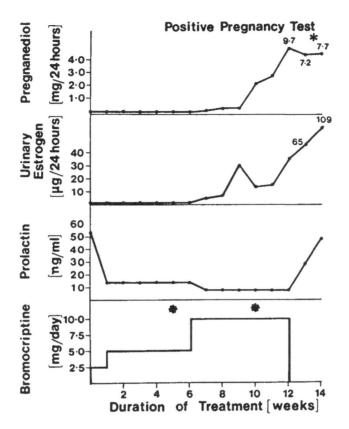

Figure 3 Weekly serum PRL and urinary estrogen and pregnanediol values in a patient who conceived following ovulation induction with bromocriptine. The asterisks in the bromocriptine panel represent the appropriate timing of PRL, estrogen and pregnanediol assays where a weekly assay program is not being used.

and the failed response comes as a complete surprise. Because of the high cost of bromocriptine and the fact that the administration of 80 mg/day is rarely much more effective than 20 mg/day in lowering PRL levels in such patients, it has been usual to reduce the maintenance dose to 20 mg/day and administer thyroxine as well, even though thyroid function has previously been shown to be normal. Theoretically the administration of thyroxine should reduce PRL levels by reducing the serum TSH levels, however, little change usually occurs in serum PRL levels during this therapy. Where a return of ovarian function still does not occur, clomiphene citrate is then given, usually in a dose of 100-150 mg/day for five days, in addition to

9

bromocriptine and thyroxine and in 6 of the 8 subjects so treated ovulation has occurred. This ovulatory response has been observed even though the serum PRL level is still mildly elevated; however it has not been observed where the serum PRL was still greater than twice the upper limit of normal.

Pregnancy following treatment with bromocriptine

It is well established that the normal pituitary enlarges during pregnancy, this enlargement being due to lactotroph cell growth consequent upon stimulation by increased estrogen levels. In addition to normal pituitary tissue, adenomatous tissue growth is also stimulated by estrogen (8) and enlargement of pituitary tumors during pregnancy, leading to optic chiasmal compression is well documented (9, 10).

The likelihood of tumor complications during pregnancies in women with previously untreated prolactinomas has been widely debated but the consensus of opinion currently is that the risk is low. Nillius et al (11), reviewing reports from 11 separate groups, found a 5.6% tumor complication rate in 146 such patients (162 pregnancies). This low complication rate suggests there is no need for potentially harmful therapy such as pituitary surgery or radiotherapy to minimize the risk of tumor growth during pregnancy, except in patients with large adenomas in whom a 35% incidence of clinically significant pituitary enlargement during pregnancy can be reduced to 7% by such therapy (10).

The current practice in Melbourne is to cease treatment with bromocriptine as soon as the pregnancy test is positive, except in patients with grade III or IV tumors, and those with grade II tumors with suprasellar extension who have not been treated surgically, where therapy is continued throughout pregnancy in the same dose used to induce ovulation. Irrespective of whether bromocriptine therapy is ceased or continued, visual field examination should be performed at least every third month during the pregnancy in order that tumor growth can be recognized early and treated appropriately. This assessment should be performed even when ther has been no evidence of a pituitary adenoma prior to pregnancy as a small tumor, too small to be recognized by the less sophisticated radiological techniques commonly used, can grow quickly and cause marked chiasmal compression.

No increase in congenital abnormalities has been identified in patients taking bromocriptine at the time of conception whether the drug was ceased as soon as a positive pregnancy test was obtained or continued throughout pregnancy (12, 13).

Treatment of Patients found to have Disordered Thyroid Function

The usual disorder of thyroid function resulting in anovulation is primary hypothyroidism. This is readily treated with thyroxine (0.1 to 0.3 mg/day) and other ovulatory stimulants are rarely required.

Where hyperthyroidism is present, this should be treated with antithyroid drugs (eg. carbimazole) and pregnancy postponed until therapy is ceased. It is unusual for the ovulatory disturbance to persist once thyroid function has been brought under control.

Treatment of Patients found to have Normal or Low FSH, LH and PRL Levels (Figure 4)

Where the patient is overweight the appropriate treatment is weight reduction as, even though ovulation induction is often achieved using clomiphene citrate, the pregnancy rate is low. During the phase of weight reduction the ovulatory disturbance commonly resolves spontaneously but if it persists when the ideal bodyweight is reached, treatment with clomiphene citrate should be given.

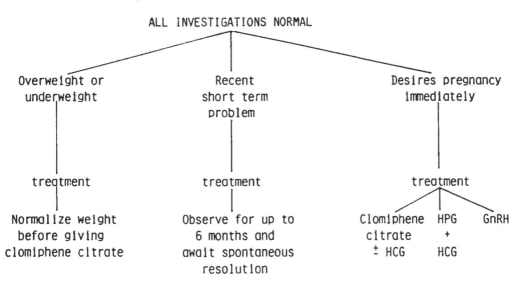

Figure 4 Management of the amenorrheic patient in whom all investigations are normal

11

Where the patient is markedly underweight (less than 85% of the ideal bodyweight), especially if other features of anorexia nervosa are present, the appropriate treatment is to increase caloric intake until the ideal bodyweight is achieved. Spontaneous ovulation usually occurs when the ideal bodyweight has been maintained for at least 12 months. Clomiphene citrate is almost always ineffective whilst the patient remains markedly underweight and for the first 6 to 12 months at ideal bodyweight, but should be tried if ideal bodyweight has been maintained for 12 months but the anovulation persists.

Where the patient is of normal weight it should not be forgotten that a significant number with oligomenorrhea and menorrhea of less than 12 months' duration (especially if the amenorrhea follows oral contraceptive administration) ovulate spontaneously and conceive during the period of investigation, presumably because of the reassurance which is provided by seeking medical assistance. This effect may be enhanced by prescribing a placebo before commencing active therapy; ovulation and pregnancy rates of 40% in patients with oligomenorrhea and 20% in patients with short term amenorrhea have been reported using placebo alone (14).

Drug treatment to induce ovulation can be with clomiphene citrate (or similar agents such as tamoxifen), gonadotropin or gonadotropin-releasing hormone (GnRH). Because of its simple mode of administration clomiphene is established as the first choice treatment for such patients with gonadotropin therapy being reserved for those who do not respond satisfactorily to treatment with clomiphene. Recently GnRH has been shown to be particularly effective in the 'clomiphene-failure' group and this treatment is likely to replace gonadotropin therapy in many such subjects. Clomiphene has proved particularly effective in cases of polycystic ovarian disease (PCOD) and in patients with some endogenous ovarian activity as indicated by a urinary estrogen excretion of >10 mcg/24 hours or those who have a progestogen induced withdrawal bleed. It is much less effective than bromocriptine in patients with elevated PRL levels.

Usual Regimen of Administration of Clomiphene

Clomiphene is usually prescribed for a five day period, generally days 5-9 or 2-6, after a spontaneous or progestogen-induced menstrual bleed. The standard starting dose is 50 mg/day but this should be reduced to 25 mg/day in patients with clinical features of PCO who may be particularly sensitive to the drug and may develop ovarian cysts on higher doses. The monitoring of therapeutic response is most often based on observation of a rise in basal body temperature of about 0.5°C between five and twelve days after completion of treatment. A more informative assessment can be obtained by mid-

tion of treatment. A more informative assessment can be obtained by mid-luteal phase measurements of progesterone in blood or pregnanediol in urine. A single luteal serum progesterone value exceeding 3 ng/ml (5) or a urinary pregnanediol value of 2 mg/24 hours or more(16) can be considered as diagnostic of an ovulatory response.

The value of a coincident estrogen measurement in the interpretation of anovulatory treatment cycles has been well documented (Table 1). A rise in estrogen without ovulation may, in the next cycle, be corrected by increasing the amount of clomiphene given or by adding mid-cycle hCG; however, when the levels of both steroids remain low a larger dose will almost always be required. Dosage increments of 50 mg/day up to a maximum of 200-250 mg/day are used if no response is obtained. Large amounts of clomiphene

Table 1 Responses to clomiphene therapy according to the day-21 urinary estrogen and preg-nanediol values, and subsequent treatment

Response to treatment	Day-21 urinary steroid excretion		Subsequent treatment
	Estrogen (mcg/24 hrs)	Pregnanediol (mg/24 hrs)	
1. Ovulation	> 20	> 2.0	Repeat treatment with same dose of clomiphene
2. Good follicular maturation ?late ovulation ?deficient corpus luteum	20-50	1.0-1.9	Repeat treatment with same dose. If same response occurs, increase dose of clomiphene
3. Good follicular response but no ovulation	50-150	> 1.0	Repeat treatment with same dose of clomiphene. Give single injection of HCG (3000-5000IU) 5-7 days after last dose of clomiphene, or when diameter of largest follicle observed on ultra-sound examination is > 19 mm
4. No significant response	< 20	< 1.0	Increase dose of clomiphene

frequently induce its commonest side-effect, hot flushes, which may restrict the ultimate dosage used.

Other unwanted effects of treatment include minor gastrointestinal symptoms, such as nausea and vomiting and abdomino-pelvic tenderness which may represent mild ovarian hyperstimulation. In the absence of endocrine monitoring, ovarian palpation is recommended at the beginning of each treatment cycle to avoid cumulative ovarian enlargement. Multiple pregnancies, usually twins, are achieved in about 10% of induced conceptions; high multiples, such as may occur with exogenous gonatropin therapy, are very rare.

Many women with hypothalamic amenorrhea will manifest a significant rise in estrogen production without ovulation and will require adjuvant hCG therapy. The timing of this single mid-cycle injection has until recently been determined empirically, usually 5-7 days after completion of clomiphene, to coincide with peak preovulatory follicular maturation(17). However, conception rates with such a regimen have proven disappointing(18). Once a mature follicle has developed, hCG (3000-5000 IU) induces ovulation within 34-40 hours of administration(19) but if it is given other than at the peak of follicular maturity, by which time adequate LH receptors have developed, hCG can cause follicular atresia and thus actively inhibit ovulation(20).

By using an ultrasonic assessment of follicular diameter it has been shown to be possible to precisely and optimally time hCG in such patients by deferring its administration until at least one follicle of 19 mm or more has developed(21). No patient required hCG before day 14 while the median day of administration was day 15; in some cycles hCG was not given until day 19. Timing of treatment in this way was almost invariably (92%) associated with ovulation and a pregnancy rate of 70% was achieved.

Results of Treatment with Clomiphene Citrate

Provided patients with ovarian failure and hyperprolactinemia are excluded, clomiphene will succeed in inducing ovulation in between about 50-80% of women with hypothalamic causes of anovulation(1,22,23). The most successful treatment subgroup is that which includes patients with relatively high basal estrogen production, in particular those with PCOD. However despite satisfactory rates of ovulation, conception rates in several series have been disappointingly low. This discrepancy between ovulation and conception rates has been ascribed to several factors, including the anti-estrogenic effects of clomiphene on cervical mucus and on the endometrium, ovum entrapment and follicular luteinization with ovulation. However, other factors must also operate because when patients who have ovulated but not

14

conceived after treatment with clomiphene citrate progress to gonadotropin therapy, their pregnancy rate is still much lower than the ovulation rate (50% compared with 96%).

The more accurate timing of ovulation using ultrasound and hCG(21) and the use of life table analysis suggest that clomiphene pregnancy rates in otherwise healthy couples are comparable with the normal spontaneous rates(24,25), though they do not approach the results achieved with exogenous gonadotropin therapy(26). A failure to achieve pregnancy within at most six ovulatory treatment cycles therefore strongly suggests that another significant antifertility factor coexists. In unsuccessfully treated patients the role of adjuvant therapy, other than preovulatory hCG, has not been established. While a definite antagonistic effect of clomiphene on mid cycle cervical mucus production has been repeatedly demonstrated, this effect is of doubtful therapeutic significance once ovulation has been satisfactorily induced. Indeed attempts to improve the mucus quality or the quantity with the administration of supplemental estrogen(27) appears to be more likely to interfere with ovulation than exert a beneficial effect(21).

Other Forms of Clomiphene Therapy

Incremental clomiphene therapy

As many as one third of patients with hypothalamic amenorrhea fail to show any increase in ovarian estrogen production when given clomiphene citrate, even when the maximum dose of 250 mg/day is given for five days. Use of clomiphene for a longer period, increasing the dose by 50 mg/day every 5 days has enabled over two-thirds of previously unresponsive patients to be ovulated successfully(28).

Twice weekly estrogen assessment was adequate during this incremental regimen to prevent ovarian hyperstimulation since clomiphene administration was stopped when estrogen values rose significantly above baseline values. Serial ultrasound examinations were then used to assess late follicular growth and to time the preovulatory hCG injection, which was almost universally required.

Ovulation was frequently induced with dosages less than the 1000 mg which had earlier failed during standard five day therapy in the same patients, suggesting that duration of exposure is as important as the amount of clomiphene given in eliciting a response.

Although it is considerably more costly than standard modes of clomiphene treatment, incremental administration remains more cost-effective and less complicated and potentially dangerous than exogenous

15

gonadotropins, hiherto the only alternative in unresponsive patients. Estrogen assays are essential, and need to be performed at least twice weekly, if hyperstimulation is to be avoided however.

Combined Clomiphene and Glucocorticoid Therapy

This combination regimen is useful in patients with elevated dehydrocpiandrosterone sulphate (DHEAS) levels who do not respond satisfactorily to treatment with clomiphene citrate alone. Dexamethasone (0.5 mg) or prednisolone (5 mg) given at night will usually suppress the DHEAS levels to normal and patients may then respond to treatment with clomiphene citrate having not done so previously.

Use of Gonadotropin Therapy for Ovulation Induction

This therapy should be reserved for patients who have not responded to treatment with clomiphene citrate or bromocriptine and pregnancy rates of up to 80% can be expected in such suitably selected patients.

In contrast to treatment with clomiphene citrate and bromocriptine, which both require an intact hypothalamus-pituitary, treatment with gonadotropin is independent of these structures and provides the total stimulus to the ovaries. Because it can act as a complete replacement, gonadotropin therapy is the most powerful and universally successful method of inducing ovulation. However, the dose requirement for FSH is critical, the difference between non-response and over-response being a dose increment of less than 50%, and the dose required by different individuals may differ by 10-fold. Before this was appreciated, hyperstimulation and multiple pregnancies with inevitable fetal loss were common.

FSH preparations are derived from human pituitaries obtained at postmortem (human pituitary gonadotropin, hPG) or from the urine of postmenopausal women (human menopausal gonadotropin, hMG). Each of these preparations is also rich in LH (FSH:LH ratio being 1:1 approximately) which ensures an adequate LH content to achieve full activity of the FSH. HPG or hMG is administered either daily or every second day, depending on the regimen chosen. When the follicle is maturing at the correct rate as assessed by urine or plasma estrogen levels, the ovulating hormone, hCG, is given. This hormone has a much longer half-life than LH and is thus more economical for clinical use.

Although theoretically a simple procedure, the treatment program with gonadotropin is most exacting as relatively small increases in the dose of gonadotropin administered can result in hyperstimulation with the production of quadruplet or quintuplet pregnancies or worse. There is no doubt that the daily injection regimen involving daily 24-hour urinary estrogen estimations to 'tailor make' the dose of gonadotropin administered(26) offers the best pregnancy rate and lowest incidence of multiple pregnancy. However, such a regimen is exceedingly demanding on both the patient and the clinician, and is expensive because of the cost of the assays required as well as th cost of the gonadotropin itself.

The principles employed in gonadotropin therapy have been described in detail previously(26,29,30) and the treatment program at the Royal Women's Hospital, devised in 1964 and reported in 1969(26), is still used today.

Initial Treatment Cycle: A base-line estrogen value is obtained three to four days before commencing treatment to ensure that the ovaries are in a quiescent phase. A starting dose of FSH is selected on the basis of her prior response to a gonadotropin stimulation test or empirically at, say, 100 iu/day. For logistic reasons, the injections are usually commenced on a Thursday and are given at 9 am daily. Complete 24 hour urine collections are commenced on the following Sunday (day four) starting at 7 to 8 am. Urinary estrogen excretion is then monitored daily, the results being available by noon. The estrogen value obtained on the Sunday to Monday urine collection (day four) determines subsequent treatment. If the estrogen value has risen rapidly and exceeds 50 mcg/24 hours, treatment is stopped and commenced later at a lower dose. If the estrogen values are rising progressively but have not reached 50 mcg/24 hours, the dose is continued. If no rise has occurred, the dose is increased on Tuesday (day six) by a factor of 1.3 and this process of incremental dosage increase every five days is continued until a rise in estrogen excretion is observed. Thus, if the starting dose is 100 iu/day, the subsequent doses are 130 iu, 170 iu, 220 iu, 285 iu and so on to a maximum of approximately 800 iu/day. It will be noted that this is a logarithmic increase. Seventy-five percent of patients respond to doses of 220 iu or less and 90% respond to doses of 400 iu or less. When a rise in estrogen excretion is observed, the daily dose of FSH being used is continued until the urinary estrogen value exceeds 50 mcg/24 hours.

The crucial decision on the further course of treatment are made when the urinary estrogen value first exceeds 50 mcg/24 hours. These decisions are complicated by the fact that the urine value obtained at noon is almost 24 hours in arrears, since it reflects the response to the previous day's injection and a further injection has already been given that morning at 8 to 9 am. Furthermore, empirical decisions may be necessary at weekends when the laboratory is closed. The rate of estrogen rise at this stage is important. If the values are rising slowly (1.1 fold/day or less) or have possibly plateaued in the region of 50 mcg/24 hours, it may be necessary to withhold treatment until the morning's estrogen value is available and, if this has not risen sufficiently, to give an additional dose of FSH at noon. If the estrogen value has risen to, say, 60 to 70 mcg/24 hours no further FSH is given and the ovulating dose of hCG is injected the following evening, 33 hours after the last dose of FSH. If the estrogen values have been rising progressively at a rate of 1.3 to 1.8 fold per day and an estrogen value exceeding 80 mcg/24 hours is expected during the 24 hour period following the last dose of FSH, the ovulating dose of hCG (3000 iu) is given 48 hours after the last dose of FSH. Although further estrogen assays cannot influence subsequent dosage administration in that cycle, urine collections and assays for estrogen and pregnanediol are continued for the six days following the ovulation dose of hCG because the pattern of response is useful for determining optimum treatment in subsequent cycles. Under correct stimulation, the estrogen values continue to rise and reach a peak of 100 to 200 mcg/24 hours on the day the hCG is given or on the next day and then fall abruptly before rising in the luteal phase. A rise in pregnanediol values during the six day period with values eventually exceeding 2.0 mg/24 hours indicates ovulation; values exceeding 4.0 mg/24 hours should be observed during supplementary treatment with hCG.

Supplementary doses of hCG are given, 100 iu on day six and 1500 iu on days 9 and 12, following the ovulating dose of hCG. The patient collects urine for estrogen and pregnanediol assays during the 24 hour periods before these injections. Occasionally these supplementary doses elicit vigorous responses, producing pregnanediol values which rapidly exceed 10 mg/24 hours; when this happens further supplementary doses are discontinued. Following completion of the supplementary doses, urine collections are continued twice weekly until pregnancy is confirmed or bleeding commences.

The Second and Succeeding Treatment Cycles: When conception has not occurred during the first cycle, treatment is commenced within the next week following onset of bleeding, provided that the estrogen and pregnanediol values have returned to the original base-line values. The doses used in the second treatment cycle depend on the responses obtained during the first. The starting dose of FSH is that which gave the successful response in the first. Once a patient's FSH requirement has been determined, it is usually reproducible from cycle to cycle. However, when in doubt the next lower dose is used and the threshold dose is approached as before by the incremental procedure. The dosage of hCG depends on the response to this hormone in the previous cycle. If ovulation occurred as judged by the occurrence of a well defined peak in estrogen excretion within three days of giving the ovulating dose of hCG, followed by an abrupt fall and then a rise associated with a rise in pregnanediol values which exceeded 2.0 mg/24 hours, the same dose of hCG is repeated.

18

If ovulation did not occur as judged by these criteria, the fault could be either in the maturation of the follicle or in the dose of hCG used. If the estrogen response as outlined in the first course of treatment was obtained (values rising continuously to exceed 50 to 60 mcg/24 hours), the ovulating dose of hCG is increased to 5000 iu in the second cycle, 7500 iu in the third, 10,000 iu in the fourth and so on until an ovulatory response is obtained. For those patients requiring 40,000 iu or more the dose is given in two equal injections at 48 and 60 hours after the last injection of FSH. Monitoring of ovarian responses and administration of supplementary doses of hCG are performed as in the first cycle of treatment. Where the ovulating dose of hCG is 10,000 iu or more, supplementary doses are not required.

If maturation of the follicle during the first course of treatment was unsatisfactory, as evidenced by a plateau of estrogen excretion at or below 50 mcg/24 hours or failure of the estrogen excretion to exceed 50 mcg/24 hours prior to the administration of hCG the ovulating dose of hCG is not increased but the dose is withheld until the estrogen levels are higher (usually 100 to 150 mcg/24 hours). Unsatisfactory follicular maturation is most commonly seen in patients with evidence of some ovarian activity prior to commencing treatment with gonadotropin and a basal urinary estrogen excretion of 20 to 30 mcg/24 hours. Increasing the dose of gonadotropin administered or continuing the same dose for a longer period will usually overcome this problem.

If follicular maturation during the initial course of treatment was excessive, as evidenced by urinary estrogen values more than doubling each day prior to the administration of hCG, the ovulating dose of hCG should not be increased even when ovulation did not occur on the previous occasion. Reduction in the dose of FSH administered will usually result in a more normal follicular response and ovulation usually results following the same dose of hCG.

Results of Treatment at the Royal Women's Hospital

The results of gonadotropin therapy using daily monitoring are illustrated in Table 2. The more severe the condition of anovulation, the better the pregnancy rate, the overall pregnancy rate being 69%. These probably represent the best conception rates possible in a specialist clinic with excellent laboratory back-up facilities. Nevertheless, even with careful monitoring the multiple pregnancy rate was almost 20%, and although the majority of these were twin pregnancies they contributed significantly to the overall fetal wastage.

19

Table 2 Results of gonadotropin therapy at the Royal Women's Hospital

	Primary amenorrhea	Secondary amenorrhea	Oligomenorrhea	Anovulatory cycles	Total
Number of women	32	142	64	5	243
Total cycles of treatment	232	776	484	56	1548
Ovulatory cycles	61%	61%	53%	55%	58%
Number who conceived	25 (78%)	105 (74%)	35 (55%)	2 (40%)	167 (69%)
Multiple pregnancy rate	11.4%	19.8%	22.2%	50.0%	19.8%
Abortion rate	12.0%	10.5%	14.3%	-	11.4%

Use of GnRH for Ovulation Induction

During the past few years several groups have reported on the therapeutic efficacy of pulsatile GnRH(31-35) and ovulation and pregnancy have been regularly achieved. These results are in contrast to the poor results observed in the early 1970's when large doses (100-150 mcg) were administered subcutaneously or intravenously thrice daily.

The mode and pattern of GnRH administration has varied but the maintenance of regular 90 minute pulses for two weeks or more has been followed by an endocrinologically normal follicular phase culminating in ovulation. It appears possible to abandon treatment after ovulation provided the luteal phase is supported with supplementary injections of hCG (1500 U) every three days until menstruation or pregnancy ensues(33). Elaborate preovulatory monitoring can also be dispensed with, since ovarian hyperstimulation is unusual and adequate information on preovulatory follicular growth can be obtained using intermittent ultrasound examination of the ovaries(36). Schoemaker et al(34) have induced ovulation with patient-administered intravenous two-hourly pulses for 16 hours per day but with the current commercial availability of small automated portable infusion pumps it seems likely that these will be most widely used to administer the GnRH. The optimal dosage of the hormone appears to vary between 10-25 mcg per pulse with the intravenous route being slightly more effective than the subcutaneous one; the latter route may be preferable in terms of patient convenience and safety however, with change of the infusion site (usually abdominal wall or inner aspect of upper arm) being necessary every four to five days. When pulses smaller than 10 mcg are used only the intravenous route is reliable(33) while doses larges than 25 mcg are likely to induce receptor desensitisation.

Pulsatile GnRH appears likely to replace exogenous gonadotropin therapy in the majority of resistant anovulatory patients with consequent distinct advantages in terms of cost, patient convenience and a lowering of multiple pregnancy rates. Hurley et al(35) reported the successful treatment of three women who had previously had high multiple pregnancies (triplets or worse) following treatment with hPG. Each conceived within two cycles of treatment with GnRH and singleton pregnancies resulted.

Despite the theoretical possibility that intrinsic feedback mechanisms would prevent hyperstimulation and multiple pregnancy during GnRH therapy, this has not been the case in clinical practice. Leyendecker(37) has already reported three multiple pregnancies - 2 sets of twins and 1 set of triplets.

GnRH has yet to be shown to be effective in disorders of ouvlation due to PCOD, in which pituitary sensitivity to GnRH is over- rather than understimulated. In this condition standard or incremental clomiphene therapy, or gonadotropin therapy, is more likely to successfully induce ovulation.

SUMMARY

Appropriate investigation has led to the recognition of 5 major endocrinological categories of anovulatory patients. The clinician is able to follow a definitive therapeutic program for each of these and, except where the FSH levels are elevated, pregnancy rates should approach values observed for normally ovulating women.

Although clomiphene citrate is likely to remain the most common drug prescribed to anovulatory women, treatment programs with clomiphene have recently been modified with much improved success rates resulting. Bromocriptine, the drug of choice for women with hyperprolactinemia, restores ovulatory cycles in most women treated, even those with pituitary tumours and usually causes tumour regression as well.

Exogenous gonadotropin therapy should be reserved for patients who do not respond to tratment with clomiphene and/or bromocriptine. With adequate monitoring the multiple pregnancy rate should be able to be kept below 20% and high-multiple pregnancies avoided. Pulsatile GnRH therapy is now replacing gonadotropin therapy for most patients who have failed to respond to clomiphene or bromocriptine, as it has distinct advantages in terms of cost, patient convenience and a lowering of multiple pregnancy rates.

REFERENCES

1. Pepperell RJ. Clinical investigation and assessment of amenorrhea, Proceedings of the 6th Asian & Oceanic Congress of Endocrinology Singapore 1978; p389
2. O'Herlihy C, Pepperell RJ, Evans JH. The significance of FSH elevation in young women with disorders of ovulation Br Med J 1980; 281:1447
3. Burrow GN, Wortzman G, Rewcastle NB, Holgate RC, Kovacs K. Microadenomas of the pituitary and abnormal sellar tomograms in an unselected autopsy series. N Eng J Med 1981; 304:156
4. Nachtigall RD, Monroe SE, Wilson CB, Jaffe RB. Prolactin-secreting pituitary adenomas in women: Absence of demonstrable adenomas in patients with altered menstrual function and abnormal sellar tomogram. Am J Obstet Gynecol 1981; 140:303
5. Pepperell RJ. Unpublished data.
6. Pepperell RJ, McBain JC, Healy DL. Ovulation induction with bromocriptine in patients with hyperprolactinemia. Aust NZ J Obstet Gynaec 1977; 17:181
7. Pepperell RJ, McBain JC, Winstone SM, Smith MA, Brown JB. Corpus luteum function in early pregnancy following ovulation induction with bromocriptine. Br J Obstet Gynaec 1977; 84:893
8. Peillon F, Villa-Porcile E, Oliver L, Racadot J. L'action des estrogenes sur les adenomes hypophysaires chez l'homme. Annals of Endocrinology (Paris) 1970; 31:259
9. Child DF, Gordon H, Mashiter K, Joplin GF. Pregnancy, prolactin and pituitary tumours. Br Med J 1975; 4:87
10. Gemzell C, Wang CF. Outcome of pregnancy in women with pituitary adenoma. Fertil Steril 1979; 31:363
11. Nillius SV, Bergh T, Larsson S-G. Pituitary tumors and pregnancy. In Pituitary Adenomas: Biology, Physiopathology and Treatment, Edited by PJ Derome, GP Hedynak, F Peillon. France, Asclepios Publishers 1980; p 103
12. Griffith RW, Turkalj I, Braun P. Outcome of pregnancy in mothers given bromocriptine. Br J Clin Pharmacol 1978; 5:227
13. Fluckiger E, del Pozo E, von Werder K. Incidence of hyperprolactinemia. In Prolactin: Physiology, Pharmacology and Clinical Findings Edited by E Fluckiger, E del Pozo, K von Werder. New York, Springer-Verlag, 1982.
14. Evans JH. The Induction of Ovulation in the Human Female (MD Thesis, University of Melbourne, 1975)
15. Israel R, Mishell DR, Stone SC, Thorneycroft IH, Moyer DL. Single luteal phse serum progesterone assay as an indicator of ouvlation. Am J Obstet Gynecol 1972; 112:1043
16. Pepperell RJ, Brown JB, Evans JH, Rennie GC, Burger HG. The investigation of ovarian function by measurement of urinary oestrogen and pregnanediol excretion. Br J Obstet Gynaec 1975; 82:32
17. Kistner RW. Use of clomiphene citrate, human chorionic gonadotropin and human menopausal gonadotropin for induction of ovulation in the human female. Fertil Steril 1966; 17:569
18. Swyer GIM, Raowanska E, McGarrigle HHG. Plasma oestradiol and progesterone estimation for the monitoring of induction of ovulation iwth clomiphene and chorionic gonadotropihin. Br J Obstet Gynaec 1976; 82:794
19. Edwards RG, Steptoe PC. Induction of follicular growth, ovulation and luteinzation in the human ovary. J Reprod Fertil (Suppl) 1975; 22:121

20. Williams RF, Hodgen GD. Disparate effects of human chorionic gonadotropin during the late follicular phase in monkeys: normal ovulation, follicular atresia, ovarian acyclicity and hypersecretion of follicle-stimulating hormone. Fertil Steril 1980; 33:64
21. O'Herlihy C, Pepperell RJ, Robinson HP. Ultrasound timing of human chorionic gonadotropin administration in clomiphene-stimulated cycles. Obst Gynecol 1982; 59:40
22. McGregor AH, Johnson JE, Bunde CA. Further clinical experience with clomiphene citrate. Fertil Steril 1968; 19:616
23. Kistner RW. Induction of ovulation with clomiphene citrate. In progress in Infertility, 2nd Edition, Edited by SJ Behrman, RW Kistner. Boston, Brown & Company, 1975, p 509
24. Gorlifsky GA, Kase NG, Speroff L. Ovulation and pregnancy rates with clomiphene citrate. Obst Gynecol 1978; 51:265
25. Hull MG, Savage PE, Jacobs HS. Investigation and treatment of amenorrhea resulting in normal fertility. B Med J 1979; 1:1257
26. Brown JB, Evans JH, Adey FD, Taft HP, Townsend L. Factors involved in the induction of fertile ovulations with human gonadotrophins. J Obstet Gynaec Brit Cwlth 1969; 76:289
27. Taubert HD, Derricks -Tan JSE. High doses of estrogens do not interfere with the ovulation- inducing effect of clomiphene citrate. Fertil Steril 1976; 27:375
28. O'Herlihy C, Pepperell RJ, Brown JB, Smith MA, Sandri L, McBain JC. Incremental clomiphene therapy: a new method for treating persistent anovulation. Obst Gynecol 1981; 58:535
29. Brown JB. Pituitary control of ovarian function - concepts derived from gonadotrophin therapy. Aust NZ J Obstet Gynaec 1978; 18:47
30. Brown BJ, Pepperell RJ, Evans JH. Disorders of ovulation. In The Infertile Couple. Edited by Pepperell, B Hudson, C Wood Edinburgh, Churchill-Livingstone, 1980, p 7.
31. Crowley WFJr, McArthur JW. Stimulation of the normal mensrual cycle in Kallman's syndrome by pulsatile administration of luteinizing-hormone releasing hormone (LHRH). J Clin Endocrinol Metab 1980; 51:173
32. Leyendecker G, Wildt L, Hansmann M. Pregnancies following chronic intermittent (pulsatile) administration of GnRH by means of a portable pump ("Zyklomat") - A new approach to the treatment of infertility in hypothalamic amenorrhea. J Clin Endocrinol Metab 1980; 51;1214
33. Reid RL, Leopold GR, Yen SSC. Induction of ovulation and pregnancy with pulsatile luteinizing hormone releasing factor: Dosage and mode of delivery. Fertil Steril 1981; 36:553
34. Schoemaker J, simons AHM, van Osnabrugge GLC, Lugtenburg C, van Kessel H. Pregnancy after prolonged pulsatile administration of luteinizing hormone-releasing hormone in a patient with clomiphene-resistant secondary amenorrhea. J Clin Endocrinol Metab 1981; 52:882
35. Hurley D, Brian R, Outch K, Stockdale J, Burger HG. Pituitary and ovarian responses to pulsatile subcutaneous gonadotrophin-releasing hormone in hypothalamic amenorrhoea: reliable ovulation and pregnancy. Proceedings of the Endocrine Society of Australia, 25th Annual Meeting, Syndey, 1982, Abstract 40.
36. O'Herlihy C, deCrespigny LJCh, Robinson HP. Monitoring ovarian follicular development with real-time ultrasound. Br J Obstet Gynaec 1980; 87:613
37. Leyendecker G, Wildt L. Induction of ovulation of GnRH in women with hypothalamic amenorrhea. J Reprod Fertil 1983; 69:397.

2

The Management of Unexplained Infertility

ERIC J THOMAS
IAN D COOKE

INTRODUCTION

It is bewildering for a patient with any medical problem to be told there is no explanation for it. This is particularly so with infertile couples because it is self-evident to them that they are not normal as they are surrounded by people who have no problem achieving pregnancy. This bewilderment is often compounded by the poor counselling that accompanies a diagnosis of unexplained infertility and the empirical prescription of treatments that are likely to cause disappointment when they fail. These two inappropriate practices probably occur because doctors are uncomfortable when they have no explanation for medical problems and tend to resort to avoidance behaviour. This results in poor counselling or the prescription of therapy in order to appear to be doing something. The final result is a disillusioned and unhappy couple who are unable to come to terms with their diagnosis or plan their future appropriately.

We feel that this approach can be improved and that the implications of a diagnosis of unexplained infertility can be openly and fully discussed with the couple. Full explanation requires information and to that end we have developed a series of investigations in both partners which further help to establish a cause for the problem. These investiations include a detailed semen analysis, ultrasonic and endocrine delineation of follicular growth and rupture and an accurately timed post-coital test and endometrial biopsy. Following this analysis of the results all the couples are counselled about alternatives ranging from acceptance of infertility, conservative management, adoption, artificial insemination by donor or in-vitro fertilisation techniques. Drug treatments are only recommended if they are aimed at a specific abnormality highlighted by the investigations. In this manner the couple obtain a full explanation of their problem and can make an educated choice about how they should proceed.

The purpose of this chapter is to describe in detail the criteria we use for a diagnosis of unexplained infertility and the further investigations offered to the patients in our research clinic. The techniques necessary for successful counselling will be reviewed as well as current treatments and their success rates.

DIAGNOSIS OF UNEXPLAINED INFERTILITY

The diagnosis of unexplained infertility depends upon the sophistication of the investigations to which the clinician has access. We believe it is reasonable to consider that a couple has unexplained infertility when the routine investigations on both partners performed by a general gynaecologist have given no diagnosis. This creates a working definition which is not only valid in Europe and North America but also in those countries who do not have ready access to complicated and expensive medical techniques. The criteria and investigations necessary for this diagnosis will now be discussed.

a) Length of Infertility

In order to be diagnosed as infertile a couple should have been practising unprotected sexual intercourse for longer than 12 months. This is based on population studies which have shown a cumulative conception rate (CCR) of 88% twelve months after cessation of contraception in apparently normal women (1, 2). The fact that in both studies 84% of the couples conceived within nine months supports the concept that normal couples should become pregnant within one year. Data from the World Health Organisation Infertility Study suggests that the frequency of sexual intecourse only affects future fertility when it is less than three times a month (3).

b) Male Partner

The cornerstone of diagnosis in the male is the semen analysis. However, examination of the external genitalia should be normal with a combined testicular volume greater than 27ml. There should be no evidence of inguinal hernia, varicocele or prostatitis and the penis should be normal with a correctly situated external urethral orifice.

Accepted parameters of a normal semen analysis have been published by the World Health Organisation (4). There are many factors which can be examined but all laboratories should be able to measure the volume of the ejaculate and sperm density, motility and morphology. In a normal semen analysis the ejaculate volume should be greater than 2ml, the sperm density greater than 20 million per ml, the rapidly progressive motility greater than 30% and the ideal morphology greater than 40%. One normal semen analysis is satisfactory to exclude a significant male factor. However the converse is not true and even fertile males frequently demonstrate abnormalities on a single semen analysis. In view of this an abnormal analysis should be repeated and the defects demonstrated to be consistent before a diagnosis of male infertility is made.

The post-coital test (PCT) has not been a routine investigation in our general infertility clinic because it is open to errors of interpretation through poor timing and observer variability. Generally a poor PCT is a reflection of an abnormal semen analysis although this is not absolute and there are

27

reports of negative PCTs in men with apparently normal semen (5). For this reason the PCT may have a role to play in further investigation of these couples and this will be discussed later.

c) Female Partner

General and gynaecological history and examination should be normal. Specifically it should be ascertained that the patient has no debilitating general disease, for example, diabetes mellitus, which would adversely affect her fertility. The 95% confidence limits for the length of the follicular phase are between 9 and 20 days (6) and for luteal phase between 12 and 17 days (7). If the two shortest and the longest intervals are combined then the normal menstrual cycle should be between 21 and 38 days although the WHO definition of regular cycles is between 25 and 35 days. Any history of intermenstrual bleeding suggests the possibility of endocrine abnormalities in the cycle - although local pathology may need to be excluded. The following investigations should all be normal.

1) Full Blood Count and Thyroid Function Tests

Both anaemia and thyroid disease affect fertility and yet they can be very difficult to diagnose clinically. In order to avoid missing a treatable cause of infertility these tests should be done as a matter of routine.

2) Plasma Prolactin

The value of this investigation is a woman without galactorrhoea who is experiencing normal menstrual cycles is debatable. However, it is possible that a mildly elevated plasma prolactin concentration may subtly interfere with either follicular growth or corpus luteum formation. In our laboratory the 97.5% confidence limit for prolactin concentration is 760 mIU/l (8). In a regularly cycling woman a single reading above this is repeated and if this is still abnormal three plasma samples are obtained during rest. Only when these samples are elevated is a diagnosis of hyperprolactinaemia made.

3) *Basal Body Temperature and Plasma Progesterone*

Each patient should measure her basal body temperature (BBT) for three cycles and a plasma progesterone sample should be obtained on Day 21 of one of these. If the pattern is biphasic and if the plasma progesterone is greater than 18 nmol/l then it is reasonable initially to assume a normal ovulatory cycle. The weakness of BBT observations is their poor capacity to differentiate normal from abnormal cycles. It is inappropriate to diagnose problems with either follicular growth, ovulation or corpus luteum formation on the BBT only. By the same token a single low plasma progesterone concentration does not necessary mean there are ovulatory abnormalities. The result should be interpreted by assessing the timing of sampling in the luteal phase from the temperature chart. It may be that Day 21 was either early or late in the luteal phase in that particular cycle in which case a low plasma progesterone would not be unexpected, so that estimation needs to be repeated. Strictly, the timing of the LH surge should be known for accurate interpretation.

4) *Hysterosalpingography*

This is the major non-invasive method by which the uterine cavity can be demonstrated allowing the diagnosis of endometrial polyps and intrauterine adhesions, which may be causing infertility, to be made. It will also give the most accurate assessment of the tubal ampullary diameter and any tubal malformations which can be difficult to diagnose laparoscopically.

5) *Laparoscopy*

Unexplained infertility can only be diagnosed after a normal laparoscopy in which the pelvis has been methodically inspected. The uterus should be inspected and any abnormality in size or shape should be noted. The length and diameter of each tube should be observed and a careful appraisal of the state of the fimbriae made. The position of any peritubal adhesions should be noted and their impact on tubal mobility assessed. Each ovary should be inspected separately including both the anterior and posterior surfaces and the fossa ovarica. This can only be done properly if a palpateur is used through a second portal. The percentage of the surface of each ovary that is covered by adhesions should be assessed as well as a percentage impact of these adhesions on ovarian mobility. Any endometriosis should be scored using the revised American Fertility Society system (9).

The pouch of Douglas, the broad ligament and the uterovesical pouch should be closely inspected for any adhesions or endometriosis. Finally the speed and ease of spill of methylene blue dye from each tube should be observed. Occasionally dye only spills from one tube in spite of the other being apparently normal. In this case the first tube should be occluded proximally with the palpateur and more dye instilled. This frequently leads to normal spill from the second tube. Unexplained infertility is only diagnosed if the pelvis is either completely normal with free spill dye bilaterally or there are adhesions which do not interfere with ovarian or tubal mobility.

In the absence of mechanical impediment to fimbrial retrieval of the oocyte, the precise relationship between infertility and asymptomatic endometriosis remains unclear. The disease is more common in infertile women and many uncontrolled trials reported high pregnancy rates after treatment. However, the only published study using a randomised non treatment control group was unable to demonstrate any benefit to future fertility from treating endometriosis (10, 11). We have performed a randomised placebo controlled trial of the treatment of asymptomatic endometriosis and demonstrated that the disease deteriorates if untreated (12). An initial analysis of the conception rate from these groups suggests that there is no benefit to future fertility from either the absence or presence of endometriosis or its successful treatment. From this we conclude that asymptomatic endometriosis should be treated but that afterwards the couple should be assumed to have unexplained infertility.

The importance of laparoscopy in the diagnosis of unexplained infertility is demonstrated by a review of 337 consecutive patients referred to our infertility clinic in 1985. Using the first four criteria discussed above 98 (29%) had unexplained infertility prior to laparoscopy. At laparoscopy 51 of these (52%) were diagnosed with endometriosis, 15 (15%) with tubal or ovarian adhesions and 32 (33%) with no demonstrable abnormality. This shows that by the correct use of common investigations only 33 (10%) out of 337 patients had unexplained infertility although this figure would increase to 84 (25%) if the patients with treated endometriosis were included.

MANAGEMENT OF UNEXPLAINED INFERTILITY

There are two explanations for the finding of unexplained infertility. The first is that the couple are normal as verified by the investigations whilst the second is that the couple are abnormal and the problem cannot be identified because of the poor sensitivity of current diagnostic techniques. Conservative management can only be justified if it is accepted that the couple is normal and as a result of that, conception will occur in time. If the second explanation is accepted then it is illogical not to investigate further or treat a couple with low fertility. In order to differentiate between normal and abnormal couples it is important to understand the relationship between length of infertility and the possibility of future pregnancy.

A cumulative conception rate is a reflection of the monthly chance of pregnancy or fecundability rate (13). The CCR from Tietze (1) and Wajntraub (2) approximate to a fecundability rate of 20%. These observations have been repeated and verified in a British population (14). However these were unselected populations which contained some infertile couples and it can be assumed that the fecundability rate in a normal population will be greater. In a study performed in Sheffield a group of apparently normal women were investigated to describe follicular growth in conception cycles and using timed intercourse, 30% became pregnant in the first cycle. This means that in normal population the fecundability rate may be as high as 30%

If a fecundability rate of 30% is translated into a CCR then 98% of that population can expect to conceive within 11 months. This interval increases to 18 months for a fecundability rate of 20% and to 37 months for a rate of 10%. Therefore after three years unexplained infertility a couple will only have a 2% chance of having a fecundability rate of 10% or greater. Even that rate is at least half and possibly a third of that of a normal population. These theoretical calculations are supported by a retrospective study of CCRs in couples with at least two years primary or secondary unexplained infertility defined by the criteria described earlier (15). After 12 months the CCR was 10% in nullipara and 18% in multipara. In a prospective study of 26 patients with unexplained infertility of a median 37 months duration the CCR at 12 months was 23% (Thomas and Cooke, unpublished data).

These CCRs reflect a maximum fecundability rate of 2% which would mean that after 24 months from diagnosis only 40% of these couples would become pregnant rising to 53% after 36 months. It can therefore be concluded that after three years infertility these couples can be assumed to be abnormal and to have a limited future fertility. As a result of these conclusions conservative management can only be justified in young couples with less that three years infertility. After that period either further investigations or treatment should be investigated. In couples with a woman over 34 years conservative management is not justified as even after two years infertility their future fertility is compromised and by waiting she may be excluded from opportunities for treatment such as in vitro fertilisation, on grounds of age alone.

Further Investigations

There are two purposes to further investigations in couples with unexplained infertility. The first is to identify a cause for the problem and the second is to provide information upon which a rational basis for further treatment can be built. Any further investigations must include a comprehensive evaluation of both the male and female partners. As a research procedure we evolved a protocol of investigations which aims to cover all diagnostic possibilities. From the outset the purpose of these investigations has been diagnostic and not therapeutic and all the couples are counselled on that basis. The protocol includes a detailed semen analysis, ultrasonic and endocrine description of follicular growth and rupture and the luteal phase, a post coital test and an endometrial biopsy. These latter two are prospectively timed with knowledge of the beginning of the mid cycle luteinizing hormone (LH) surge. Table 1 shows the timing occurring on Day 14 and from this it can be seen that the protocol provides an accurate and comprehensive description of both male and female. The individual investigations will now be analysed in detail.

a) *Ultrasound*

The use of ultrasound to visualise and measure the developing follicle has added a new dimension to the diagnosis of abnormalities in folliculogenesis. We use a Combison 320 mechanical sector scanner with a 3 mHz probe (Kretztechnik). The follicle appears as an intra-ovarian echo-free cyst which is identifiable from approximately seven days before the LH surge. Initially there are a number of small follicles visible but the dominant follicle becomes obvious once it has achieved a diameter of 5-7 mm and the rest undergo atresia. An initial scan is performed firstly to identify any abnormalities such as follicular or endometrial cysts which may have appeared since the normal laparoscopy. The second reason for performing this scan is to observe the ovaries for peripherally situated micro-cysts in polycystic ovary syndrome which can occur in normally cycling women (16, 17). Scanning is performed daily once a dominant follicle has been identified.

The follicular diameter is measured in the vertical and horizontal planes on three occasions and the volume is calculated from means of these. If the follicle is assumed to be a sphere we have demonstrated a good correlation between actual and calculated volume ($r = 0.861$; $n = 43$). Follicular rupture is diagnosed by the disappearance of the follicle or a marked decrease in size. The appearance of a fluid track from the ovary or of fluid in the pouch of Douglas are used as confirmatory evidence (19). Further evidence can be obtained by observing the endometrium for the appearance of an 'ovulation ring' (20). However care must be employed in using this observation as it probably reflects alterations in the endocrine environment and does not verify follicular rupture.

If the follicle ruptures then ultrasonography is continued for a further two days until corpus luteum formation is observed. If there is no rupture the scanning is continued until the follicle shows definite cyst formation or is no longer an entity that can be measured accurately. It is observed for loss of demarcation of the wall and the appearance of intra-follicular echoes which are signs of in-situ luteinization (21). We have not been able to observe pre-ovulatory changes within the follicle although some investigators claim to be able to visualise the appearance of the cumulus oophorous after the beginning of the LH surge (22).

The difficulty with using ultrasound to diagnose abnormal follicular growth is that there is limited evidence of what constitutes a normal pattern. Several studies have reported the growth patterns in spontaneous cycles in normal volunteers (23, 24, 25). They all report that the follicle can be measured from six days before the LH surge and follows a linear increase in volume from then. However, the range of mean preovulatory volumes ranges from 1.1 to 8.7 ml. This large range probably represents variability between different observers and different ultrasound machines. Only one study has observed follicular growth in spontaneous conception cycles and reported a linear increase in volume with mean pre-ovulatory value of 3.9 ml (26). A similar study in our department (Lenton, EA, unpublished observations) has demonstrated similar results. We have therefore defined normal follicular growth as a linear increase in volume up to minimum value of 2.0 ml on the day of the LH surge.

The mean interval from the beginning of the LH surge to follicular rupture is 32 hours (27). A follicle can either rupture appropriately, prematurely or remain unruptured. Premature follicular rupture occurs within 24 hours of the LH surge and should be accompanied by the observation of fluid in the pouch of Douglas to differentiate it from follicular atresia. Delayed rupture is diagnosed if the follicle remains intact for longer than 48 hours after the beginning of the LH surge. Whether the resultant structure is designated as a follicular cyst, a luteal cyst or a luteinized unruptured follicle depends on an integration of plasma or salivary progesterone concetrations representing the luteal phase growth pattern to evaluate its endocrine function.

b) *Plasma Gonadotropins*

Two blood samples are taken in the early follicular phase for estimation of luteinising hormone (LH) and follicle stimulating hormone (FSH) concentrations. From Day 7 onwards the samples are taken daily in order to document precisely the timing and synchrony of the mid-cycle gonadotropin surge with plasma oestradiol concentration and follicular growth and rupture. The normal values for plasma LH, FSH, and oestradiol in conception cycles have already been published (8). The two samples in the early follicular phase are taken to document the ratio between the concentrations of LH and FSH as this is the time when both are most constant. Later in the follicular phase the concentration of FSH drops and then both gonadotropins rise as part of the mid-cycle surge. An LH to FSH ratio of greater than 3:1 in two separate samples is considered abnormal and probably represents a type of polycystic ovary syndrome in spite of regular cycles. Any woman with a high LH/FSH ratio has the plasma concentration of testosterone, androstenedione and sex hormone binding concentration measured in order to diagnose any abnormalities in androgen secretion or carriage.

c) *Plasma Oestradiol*

This is sampled daily throughout the second half of the follicular phase, the peri- and post-ovulatory period. Plasma concentrations should demonstrate an increase from approximately six days before the LH surge and peak one day before it. In conception cycles this peak exceeds 400 pmol/l (8) and this is defined as the lower limit of normal. A follicle can only be described as normal if both the physical growth as described by ultrasound and the endocrine function as described by plasma oestradiol are normal.

d) *Salivary Progesterone*

In the past one of the major difficulties about performing detailed studies of the menstrual cycle has been the necessity for daily plasma sampling throughout which has greatly decreased patient compliance. Recent work has shown that salivary and plasma progesterone concentrations correlate well in both normal and abnormal luteal phases (28, 29). It is considered that the transfer of progesterone from plasma to saliva is rapid and analagous to ultrafiltration but precisely what mechanism is employed is unknown (30).

There is no apparent circadian rhythm in salivary progesterone concentration and no degradation of the hormone if the sample is allowed to stand for up to three days at room temperature (31). These authors concluded that it was entirely satisfactory for patients to store the samples at home in a domestic freezer. This recommendation means that a daily estimation of progesterone concentration can be made without the patient being required to attend the clinic. Each patient is issued with a box containing 35 plastic containers into which she expectorates 2.5 ml of saliva each day throughout the cycle. The saliva is stored in her own freezer and all samples returned to the clinic within one week of menstruation. We have found excellent compliance with this method which allows a detailed description of not only the adequacy of the luteal phase but also of any occurrence of premature luteinization of a pre-ovulatory follicle. The progesterone concentrations are measured by direct radioimmunoassay using a method similar to that described by Chearshul et al (1982) (32).

The range of peak salivary concentrations in the normal luteal phase is between 300 and 600 pmol/l (29, 31). Both these studies measured salivary progesterone in conception cycles and showed that it mirrored the concentrations in the first half of normal luteal phases. We have verified the same pattern in spontaneous conception cycles investigated in this department (Lenton E A, unpublished observations). A normal luteal phase is, therefore, defined as one of between 12 and 17 days in which the daily salivary progesterone concentrations exceed 300 pmol/l consistently between five and eight days after the LH surge.

c) *The Post-Coital Test and Endometrial Biopsy*

The accuracy of the information from both the post-coital test (PCT) and an endometrial biopsy depend absolutely on the correct timing of the observation in relation to the LH surge. This is because this powerful endocrine signal initiates the alterations in ovarian steroid hormone secretion which radically alter both cervical mucus and the endometrium. In order to time these observations correctly we use the recently developed monoclonal antibody LH urinary dipsticks ('Ovusticks' Monoclonal Antibodies, Oxford) to accurately determine the onset of the LH surge. Once the follicle has attained a diameter of 14 mm the patients collect their urine daily and bring this sample to the clinic every morning where it is tested with a dipstick. An increasing urinary LH concentration is signalled by a colour change and thus the start of the LH surge can be immediately determined. The PCT is performed 24 hours after and the endometrial biopsy seven days after the beginning of the LH surge.

The PCT is performed 6 to 10 hours after intercourse in the manner described in the new WHO laboratory manual. The Insler score if used to describe the quality of the cervical mucus and a normal PCT is defined as at least ten progressively motile sperm per high power field (X400). An abnormal PCT is repeated in a subsequent cycle and if the result is the same then by comparing it with the detailed semen analysis (qv), the Insler score and the detailed endocrine results it can be determined whether the problem rests in the male, an abnormal cervical mucus or as a result of hormonal abnormalities or antibody production in the female.

The endometrial biopsy is performed as an outpatient procedure with a Sharman curette which requires either no or minimal cervical dilatation. The procedure is virtually painless and gives an excellent biopsy from the anterior uterine wall. The endometrium is dated using the histological criteria of Noyes, Hertig and Rock (33). The result is described as normal if the blind histological dating is within two days of the actual time of biopsy. An abnormal result is compared with the salivary progesterone concentrations in the luteal phase and it can thus be concluded whether there is a primary endometrial abnormality or the appearances are secondary to hormonal dysfunction.

d) *Semen Analysis*

The purpose of the semen analysis is to investigate sperm characteristics in more detail than can be done in a routine infertility clinic. The sample is collected by masturbation after three days abstention and ejaculate volume and sperm density are measured in the same way as in a routine analysis. pH is assessed using an electrode. A differential assessment of motility is performed and the sperm are described as that percentage which is rapidly progressively motile, moderately progressively motile, motile with no progression and immotile. A careful assessment of morphology is undertaken with the sperm being categorised as ideal or as having defects of the head, tail or neck. Some examples of these would be small heads, large heads, two tails and broken necks.

Seminal adenosine triphosphate is measured using the method described by Comhaire et al (34). The purpose of this is to give an indication of the energy potential of the sperm. A mixed antiglobulin reaction test is performed using either sensitised human red blood cells in the manner described by Cerasaro et al (35) or an immunobead test. If over 10% of the sperm have adherent cells or latex particles then there is evidence of autoantibodies deposited on the sperm. Finally a peroxidase stain is used to differentiate sperm precursors from leucocytes which take up the stain as the two appear very similar on light microscopy.

A seminal abnormality is only diagnosed if the defect is consistent in two consecutive analysis. In this technique semen is placed in a test tube and covered with a buffer solution. After 60 to 90 minutes those sperms which have migrated to the surface or 'swum up', are analysed for density and differential motility. This gives a further impression of sperm motility and because this technique is necessary for capacitation and selection of sperm for in-vitro fertilisation it enables a prognosis to be made for this mode of treatment for male factor infertility.

Many couples with unexplained infertility have experienced protracted delays between investigation and therefore this protocol is designed to be completed within one menstrual cycle. This will be extended to the middle of the next cycle if either the semen analysis or PCT needs to be repeated. Analysis of the results takes approximately eight weeks so that the couple are seen for counselling about the findings within three to four months of starting the cycle to be studied. Over 300 couples have undergone a variation of this protocol and some initial results have already been reported (36). We expect to reveal a significant male or female factor in approximately four out of five couples. The broad diagnostic categories are abnormalities in:

1) Semen analysis
2) Follicular growth and endocrine function
3) Follicular rupture
4) Gonadotropin secretion
5) Corpus luteum function
6) Endometrial function
7) Cervical mucus

Many couples have more than one abnormality which may be entirely separate or interdependent. For example, problems with follicular rupture may be either primary or secondary to abnormal gonadotrophin secretion and in the same manner corpus luteum dysfunction may be primary or secondary to follicular abnormalities. The great benefit of the protocol of investigations is that it is comprehensive enough to allow these relationships to be revealed and hence the primary problem diagnosed. Data on the reproducibility of the endocrine findings are available (37), although the variability in follicle data is likely to be greater. Nevertheless this approach is practical and awaits a better one.

TREATMENT OF UNEXPLAINED INFERTILITY

The history of medicine repeatedly shows that the treatment of any disorder is usually ineffective until its cause has been elucidated. We, therefore, believe that the most important development in the management of unexplained infertility is the introduction of comprehensive diagnostic techniques and hence we have developed the protocol of investigations described earlier. Each couple is counselled with the results and the benefits of therapy against alternatives such as acceptance of infertility or adoption discussed. This counselling will be explored in greater detail later in the chapter. At the moment the main treatment options are donor insemination (AID) or in vitro fertilisation (IVF) for the male and drug therapy, IVF or gamete intra-fallopian transfer for the female.

a) **Male Problems**

It is surprising how often a detailed semen analysis will highlight previously undiagnosed abnormalities. The severity of these defects, the length of infertility and the absence or presence of female factors all influence the recommendation of treatment. If a seminal defect is the sole abnormality and our investigations reveal a normal female then after three to four years of infertility the chance of spontaneous conception is low. In these cases AID should be presented as the best treatment. If the abnormality is asthenozoospermia from which there is a successful migration then IVF should be considered. However, it should be noted that sperm abnormalities are likely to be a manifestation of major functional problems and that fertilisation rates are likely to be severely reduced. IVF may well be the treatment of choice if there are both male and female problems as it may overcome both. Finally the intrauterine insemination of prepared husband's semen (AIH) is an ineffective treatment for male factor infertility if the females are rigorously shown to be normal (38) and therefore there is no logic to using it in unexplained infertility.

b) **Drug Therapy**

There is no place for the unselected and empirical prescription of ovulation induction therapy, such as clomiphene, in the treatment of unexplained infertility especially as no data exist to show that such intervention is beneficial. Therapy should only be recommended to overcome a specific defect in the menstrual cycle. We prescribe clomiphene to these women who have poor follicular growth with low oestradiol secretion in whom there are no abnormalities of follicular rupture or gonadotropin secretion. In those women with abnormal LH:FSH ratios with abnormal androgen concentrations, the adrenal production of testosterone and androstenedione are suppressed with dexamethasone. Progestin support for the luteal phase is used only in those women in whom corpus luteum dysfunction is a primary problem and not secondary to poor follicular growth or abnormalities in the gonadotrophins. Often the study of the menstrual cycle is repeated whilst the patient is on treatment to prove that it has had a beneficial impact. It is only by combining such careful monitoring with prescription for defined defects alone that drug therapy can be assessed as having any benefit in unexplained infertility.

c) IVF and GIFT

IVF and recently GIFT have both been reported as treatments for unexplained infertility with varying rates of success. These techniques may work by overcoming the abnormality that is causing the infertility or, because multiple embryo transfer occurs, they may simply increase the fecundability rate in that cycle. The success rates of IVF in unexplained infertility equate with a simple increase in fecundability rate by a factor of three or four because of multiple embryo transfer.

GIFT is a recently developed technique (39) and pregnancy rates of up to 35% per cycle have been reported in patients with unexplained infertility (40). This far exceeds the expected rate of 8-10% if the success were simply an increase in fecundability rate and suggests that GIFT may be overcoming a major problem. Logically this must be abnormalities of oocyte retrieval either because of an intrinsic fimbrial defect or because of unruptured follicles. At the moment the evidence is from only small numbers of patients and further large studies are needed as well a a close inspection of diagnostic criteria for unexplained infertility and of pregnancy. However, even with these reservations, GIFT appears to be an interesting innovation in the treatment of unexplained infertility.

FUTURE DEVELOPMENTS

The technique of follicular aspiration for the purposes of IVF has provided opportunities for observation of the morphology of the oocyte, the intrafollicular steroid environment and the interaction between the sperm and the oocyte in couples with unexplained infertility. Unfortunately, hyperstimulation regimes mask the normal physiological state and it is not possible to correlate any of these parameters except sperm-oocyte interaction with a cause of infertility. In order to overcome this we aspirate the follicle in unstimulated cycles, using the transvesical technique described by

Lenz and Lauritson (41), 28 to 36 hours after the spontaneous LH surge as documented by dipsticks. This is combined with the intensive ultrasonic and endocrine monitoring previously described.

Following aspiration the morphology of the oocyte and cumulus oophorus is described and the follicular fluid frozen for future analysis. The oocyte is incubated with sperm and both fertilisation and embyro growth observed. If the latter is normal then the embryo is replaced at the four cell stage. At a later date the follicular fluid is assayed for concentrations of oestradiol, progesterone, androgens and LH. In this way it is possible to correlate the intrafollicular environment with oocyte normality and capacity to fertilise and grow as a normal embryo. It provides a rigorous definition of normality in the female which means that in these cases failure to fetilise must be due to abnormalities in the sperm. At the moment the data are preliminary and we are still defining the limits of normality but in the future this technique has great potential for increasing diagnostic capabilities.

COUNSELLING

Throughout this chapter the importance of counselling has been stressed. It is our experience that these couples are able to understand quite complex endocrine concepts if properly explained and respond well to open and informed discussion. In the final analysis the decision to continue further investigations or treatment rests with the couple and is a reflection of their past experience and future expectations of their lifestyle. In order for them to make this decision and be able to come to terms with it they must be realistically advised as to their future possibilities of conception. It is counter productive for the clinician to attempt to disguise any areas of general or personal ignorance. With very few exceptions we have found this counselling technique to have been well received by the patients. Of course the information provided by the detailed investigation makes counselling much more straightforward. In fact the only advice that these couples do not respond to is that they have nothing wrong with them and there is no need to worry.

CONCLUSION

Unexplained infertility is a perplexing disorder for the couple which will only be resolved by careful and logical investigation or its cause. We have described the protocol used in our clinic and present it as a framework for future development. Naturally it is not completely adequate but it attempts to fulfill the basic necessity in the management of unexplained infertility which is that diagnosis should precede treatment.

REFERENCES

1. Tietze C. Fertility after discontinuation of intrauterine and oral contraception. Int J Fertil 1968; 13:386-389
2. Wajntraub G. Fertility after removal of the intrauterine ring. Fertil Steril 1970; 21:555-557
3. Cooke I D. Results from the female partner. Abstract 17, 12th World Congress on Fertility & Sterility, Singapore (1986)
4. Belsey M A, Eliasson R, Gallegos A J, Moghissi K, Paulsen C and Prasad M. Laboratory manual for the examination of human semen and semen-cervical mucus interaction. Press Concern, Singapore 1980
5. Schats R, Aitken R J, Templeton A A and Djahanbakch O. The role of cervical mucus-semen interaction in infertility of unknown aetiology. Br J Obstet Gynaecol 1984; 91:371-376
6. Lenton E A, Landgren B-M and Sexton L. Normal variation in the length of the luteal phase of the menstrual cycle: identification of the short luteal phase. Br J Obstet gynaecol 1984; 91:685-689
7. Lenton E A, Landgren B-M, Sexton L and Harper R. Normal vairation in the length of the follicular phase of the menstrual cycle: effect of chronological age. Br J Obstet gynaecol 1984; 91:681-684
8. Lenton E A, Sulaiman R, Sobowale O and Cooke I D. The human menstrual cycle: plasma concentrations of prolactin, LH, FSH, oestradiol and progesterone in conceiving and non conceiving women. J Reprod Fert 1982; 65:131-139
9. American Fertility Society. Revised American Fertility Society Classification of Endometriosis. Fertil Steril 1985; 43:351-352
10. Seibel M M, Berger M J, Weinstein F G and Taymor M L. The effectiveness of danazol on subsequent fertility in minimal endometriosis. Fertil Steril 1982; 38:534-537
11. Bayer S, Seibel M, Suffan D, Berger M and Taymor M. The efficacy of danazol treatment in an infertile population with mild endometriosis. Abstract 47, 42nd Annual Meeting of the American Fertility Society, Toronto, Canada, 1986
12. Thomas E J and Cooke I D. The impact of gestrinone upon the natural history of endometriosis. Br Med J 1987; 294:272-274
13. Cooke I D, Sulaiman R A, Lenton E A and Parsons R J. Fertility and infertility statistics: Their importance and application. Clin Obstet Gynaecol 1981; 8:531-548
14. Vessey M P, Wright N H, McPherson K and Wiggins P. Fertility after stopping different methods of contraception. Br Med J 1978; 276:265-267
15. Lenton E A, Weston G A and Cooke I D. Long-term follow up of the apparently normal couple with a complaint of infertility. Fertil Steril 1977; 28:913-919
16. Franks S, Adams J, Mason H and Polson D. Ovulatory disorders in women with polycystic ovary syndrome. Clin Obstet Gynaecol 1985; 12:605-632
17. Adams J, Polson D W and Franks S. Prevalence of polycystic ovaries in women with anovulation and idiopathic hirsutism. Br Med J 1986; 293:355-359
18. Nitschke-Dabelstein S, Hackeloer B J and Sturm G. Ovulation and corpus luteum formation observed by ultrasonography. Ultrasound in Medicine and Biology 1981; 7:33-39
19. de Crespigny L Ch, O'Herlihy C and Robinson H P. Ultrasonic observation of the mechanism of human ovulation. Am J Obstet Gynecol 1981; 139:636-639
20. Hackeloer B J and Sallam H N. Ultrasound scanning of ovarian follicles. Clin Obstet Gynaecol 1983; 10:603-620
21. Coulam C B, Hill L M and Breckle R. Ultrasonic evidence for luteinzation of unruptured preovulatory follicles. Fertil Steril 1982; 37:524-529
22. Goswamy R K, Williams G, Howles C, Macnamee M, Edwards R G and Steptoe P C. A comparison of abdominal mechanical sector ultrasound with vaginal mechanical sector ultrasound in monitoring follicular growth and development during natural and clomid cycles. 18th Annual Meeting of the British Medical Ultrasound Society, Conventry, December 1986

23. Ylostalo, Ronnberg L and Jouppila P. Measurement of the ovarian follicle by ultrasound in ovulation induction. Fertil Steril 1979; 31:651-655
24. O'Herlihy C, de Crespigny L Ch, Lopata A, Johnson I, Hoult I and Robinson H. Pre-ovulatory follicular size: a comparison of ultrasound and laparoscopic measurements. Fertil Steril 1980; 34:24-26
25. Smith D H, Picher R H, Sinosich M and Saunders D M. Assessment of ovulation by ultrasound and estradiol levels during spontaneous and induced cycles. Fertil Steril 1980; 33:387-390
26. Zegers-Hochschild F, Lira G G, Paracha M and Lorengi E A. A comparative study of the follicular growth profile in conception and non-conception cycles. Fertil Steril 1984; 41:244-247
27. Edwards R G, Steptoe P C, Fowler R E and Baillie J. Observations on preovulatory human ovarina follicles and their aspirates. Br J Obstet Gynaecol 1980; 87:769-779
28. Choe J K, Khan-Dawood F S and Dawood M Y. Progesterone and estradiol in the saliva and plasma during the menstrual cycle. Am J Obstet Gynecol 1983; 147:557-562
29. Zorn J R, McDonough P G, Nessman C, Janssens Y and Cedard L. Salivary progesterone as an index of luteal function. Fertil Steril 1984; 41:248-253
30. Riad-Fahmy D, Read G F, Walker R G and Griffiths K. Steroids in saliva for assessing endocrine function. Endocrine Reviews 1982; 3:367-395
31. Walker S M, Walker R F and Riad-Fahmy D. Longitudinal studies of luteal function by salivary progesterone determinations. Hormone Res 1984; 20:231-240
32. Chearskul S, Ricon-Rodriguez I, Sufi S B, Donaldson A and Jeffcoate S L. Simple direct assays for measuring estradiol and progesterone in saliva. In: Radioimmunoassay and Related Procedures, International Atomic Energy Authority, Vienna, 1982, pp 265-274
33. Noyes R W, Hertig A T and Rock J. Dating the endometrial biopsy. Fertil Steril 1950; 1:3
34. Comhaire F, Vermeulen L, Ghedira K, Mas J, Irvine S and Gallipolis G. Adenosine triphosphate in human semen a quantitative estimate of fertilizing potential. Fertil Steril 1983; 40:500-504
35. Cerasaro M, Valenti M, Massacesi A, Lenzi A and Dondero F. Correlation between the direct IgG MAR test (mixed antiglobulin reaction test) and seminal analysis in men from infertile couples. Fertil Steril 1985; 44:390-395
36. Lenton E A. Simultaneous ovarian ultrasonography and endocrine monitoring in women with unexplained infertility. Abstract 296, 11th Meeting of Internation Federation of Fertility Societies, Dublin 1983
37. Lenton E A, Lawrence G F, Coleman R A and Cooke I D. Individual variation in gonadotrophin and steroid concentrations in the lengths of the follicular and luteal phases in women with regular menstrual cycles. Clin Reprod Fertil 1983; 2:143-150
38. Thomas E J, McTighe L, King H, Lenton E A, Harper R and Cooke I D. Failure of high intrauterine insemination of husband's semen. Lancet 1986; ii:693-694
39. Asch R H, Ellsworth L R, Balmaceda J P and Wong P C. Pregnancy after translaparoscopic gamete intrafallopian transfer. Lancet 1984; ii:1034-1035
40. Yovich J L, Matson P I, Turnon S R, Richardson P A and Blacklodge D. Pregnancy rates in a gamete intra-fallopian transfer (GIFT) program are markedly affected by semen quality. Abstract 742, 12th World Congress on Fertility & Sterility Singapore (1986)
41. Lenz S and Lauritson J G. Ultrasonocially guided percutaneous aspiration of human follicles under local anaesthesia: a new method of collecting oocytes for in vitro fertilization. Fertil Steril 1982; 38:673-677

3

Laser Surgery for Infertility: Past, Present and Future

WILLIAM R KEYE, Jr

INTRODUCTION

In spite of the fact that lasers have been used in gynecology for nearly a decade, there is still an active debate over their role and value. At present even laser surgeons are divided in their choice of wavelengths, delivery system, and adjunctive therapy. Consequently, gynecologists without laser experience are often confused and undecided about the value of the laser in their own practice. A review of the past, present, and future of lasers in gynaecology may assist the clinical gynecologist in deciding whether or not to learn about the use of lasers in his or her infertility practice.

PAST AND PRESENT

The first report of gynecologic laser surgery by Bellina in 1974 followed the use of lasers in several other medical specialities (1). Since that time, numerous investigators have reported the application of several different wavelengths for the treatment of disorders of the uterus, fallopian tubes, and ovaries.

The first application of lasers to the treatment of infertility-related pathology involved the CO_2 laser to lyse peritubal adhesions and open obstructed fallopian tubes at laparotomy(2,3).

About the same time Bruhat of France and Tadir of Israel described the delivery of the laser through the laparoscope(4.5). Initially they used the CO_2 laser laparoscopy for tubal sterilization but soon abandoned laser sterilization because of the unacceptably high rate of tubal recanalization. Since these initial reports, however, several investigators and clinicians in this country have reported the safe and effective use of the CO_2 laser through the laparoscope in the treatment of pelvic adhesions, hydrosalpinges, endometriosis, and polycystic ovaries(6-13).

Currently, the CO_2 laser is used at laparoscopy and laparotomy for the treatment of many types of infertility-related pathology including endometriosis, tubal obstructions, peritubal adhesions, polycystic ovary syndrome, uterine myomata, uterine septae, and ooclusive periovarian adhesions. The clinical results appear to be at least as good as standard microsurgical techniques. In addition, the laser has facilitated the laparoscopic treatment of many forms of pelvic pathology, thus reducing cost, morbidity, and recovery time.

In 1983 Keye reported his initial experience with the argon laser for the treatment of endometriosis(14). He selected the argon laser because of the selective absorption by the hemosiderin-stained endometriotic implants of the argon laser wavelength (488nm) and the ability to deliver the argon laser

44

energy through a flexible wave guide. After experiments on induced endometriosis in rabbits, he treated over 250 women with mild or moderate endometriosis. He recently reported a 68% pregnancy rate among women with endometriosis and infertility of short duration (<2 years)(15). Keye also reported the vaporization of periovarian and peritubal adhesions secondary to endometriosis.

The argon laser offers the advantages of selective damage of the implants with little or no damage to surrounding or underlying tissues and minimal chance of perforation of bowel or bladder. In addition, the ability to deliver the argon laser through flexible fiber facilitates the lysis of adhesions and coagulation or vaporization of endometriotic implants behind the ovary.

Lamano reported the use of the Nd:YAG for the laparoscopic treatment of endometriosis(16). While the Nd:YAG laser coagulates rather than vaporizes the implants, the thermal effect of this laser occurs below the surface and is not specific for the pigmented lesions of endometriosis. In spite of these disadvantages, Lamano reported safe and effective treatment of mild and moderate endometriosis with the use of the Nd:YAG laser.

Keye and co-workers recently performed studies in animals and humans with the Nd:YAG laser and quartz fiber coupled to a sapphire-contact laser probe(17). When delivered through the sapphire tip, the Nd:YAG laser will cut and excise as well as coagulate. This combination of Nd:YAG laser and contact probe combines the advantages of the CO_2 laser (vaporization and surface effect) with those of the Nd:YAG laser (delivery through a flexible fiber and coagulation of larger blood vessels).

Reports by Goldrath et al demonstrated a role of the Nd:YAG laser in the treatment of endometrial pathology via the hysteroscope(18). They reported the creation of an Asherman's syndrome in women with abnormal uterine bleeding who were not good candidates for hysterectomy. Recently, Goldrath also used the Nd:YAG laser and the hysteroscope to photocoagulate submucosal myomas, uterine septae and intrauterine adhesions. To date, the results are too preliminary to draw any conclusions regarding the long-term efficacy and safety of such therapy.

A recent addition to the array of lasers for gynecologic surgery is the KTP-532 (potassium-titanyl-phospate 532nm) laser. This experimental laser, which creates a laser beam with many of the tissue effects of the argon laser, has been used to treat endometriosis and other pelvic pathology with some initial success in a small number of patients(19,20). The disadvantage of the KTP-532 laser is its expense, limited power, and investigational status.

The limitation of the currently available lasers is the fact that all of them deliver a single wavelength over a relatively narrow range of power. In all probability the future of lasers in the treatment of infertility will necessitate tunable lasers which are capable of delivering a wide range of wavelengths.

FUTURE

A number of variable wavelength lasers have been developed. These tunable lasers can be divided into three categories according to wavelength: (1) less than 200nm, (2) between 200nm and 25 micrometers and (3) between 25 micrometers and 1mm. Presently, there is no single source that exists which can, as a single laser, deliver laser energy continuously over this entire range. However, there are several lasers such as the dye laser that can operate in a tunable fashion over parts of this range. The dye laser is tunable over a range of 350 to 1100nm but is capable of delivering power only in the range of a few watts.

There has been a concerted effort to develop a variable wavelength laser that is not only efficient and powerful but will have the capacity to deliver a wide range of frequencies that can be tuned continuously to match absorption characteristics of the absorbing tissues. The results of these efforts is the free electron laser (FEL) which satisfies these criteria.

The free electron laser creates a high-energy electron beam which passes through a tunable magnetic field called a "wiggler" or "undulator". The "wiggler" consists of a series of magnets which are lined up so that their polarity alternates. The magnetic field that is created forces the electrons in the beam to oscillate in a transverse direction and to emit a laser beam in the forward direction. If this laser beam is propagated colinearly with the electron beam there is an interaction between the two beams with the transfer of energy from the electron beam to the laser beam. Under specific conditions, this transfer of energy can create an amplification of the laser beam. The wavelength of the resultant laser beam can be tuned by varying the beam velocity and/or the magnetic field strength.

While there are no theoretical limits to the wavelengths that can be produced, there are practical limits imposed by technological considerations such as beam current, optic quality, and achievable magnetic field strength and periodicity. Free electron lasers have the capability of operating as powerful sources of continuously tunable, coherent radiation in wavelengths ranging from the far-infrared to the far-ultraviolet.

The term, "free electron laser," was termed by John Madey of Stanford, who headed a group that built the first laser in 1976. Advances in the past decade have led to a second generation of FEL's and hopes of additional generations of FEL's with the following characteristics:

1. Efficiency - 10% to 20%
2. Power - 10kW to 1MW
3. Wavelength - 50nm to (10)6 nm (1mm)
4. Pulse length - 10^{-12} to infinity

An example of a FEL currently in operation is the one at Stanford, which is only 15 feet with a laser head only seven feet long. This FEL is tunable from a wavelength of 11 micrometers to 2 micrometers simply by varying the spacing of the magnets. The output of this laser consists of pulses that are 2 to 8 picoseconds in duration, with peak powers of 10 megawatts (average power of 100 watts) spaced 30 pico seconds apart. Additional programs are being planned which will include strong biomedical components.

Free electron lasers will have biomedical, as well as non-medical applications. Notable among the non-biomedical applications are its use in spectroscopic studies of semi-conductors and other solids, gases and liquids in the field of surface chemistry and as a high energy anti-missile military weapon.

Because of the unique properties of the FEL, many of the biomedical applications of the free electron laser are not a direct or obvious extension of present laser uses. Biomedical applications of the FEL wil include both basic and clinical studies. Basic research with the free electron laser will include more detailed studies of the effects of many wavelengths on tissue, including the early effects of laser light on macro-molecular changes in living cells, a redefining of the threshold for laser-induced tissue injury, and the study of changes in blood flow induced by laser energy. In addition to these basic studies of laser biology, there are a number of potential clinical applications. Some of these are described below.

1. **Accelerated Wound Healing** - The recent observation of increased strength of skin wounds exposed to low intensity 632.8 He-Ne light and its impact on the rate of collagen synthesis by fibroblasts suggest the application of other wavelengths to the study of wound healing. It has been postulated that there are wavelengths that can modify enzyme structure or function and, as a result, protein synthesis, energy metabolism, and the synthesis of other critical cellular biomolecules such as DNA and RNA. It is hoped that such studies will lead to the use of lasers to accelerate wound healing.

2. **Photodynamic Tumour Destruction** - One of the exciting new developments in the medical application of lasers has been the use of 532 nm radiation from the argon-pumped rhodamine B dye laser to photodynamically activate hematoporphyrin derivatives. However, there are limitations of this system in the treatment of very large tumours because of the limited power output of these dye lasers (maximum output of four watts). It is possible that radiation in the range of 10 to 20 watts would allow the treatment of significantly larger tumours and large tumour beds. Such treatments may well be sufficiently fast and efficient to allow photodynamic therapy to be used intraoperatively to irradiate a tumour bed and its regional lymphatics and thus destroy metastasizing cells. In addition, the availability of new

wavelengths will undoubtedly lead to the development of new dyes for photodynamic therapy, making it possible to treat larger tumours or tumours located below the surface of tissues and organs. In addition, it may be possible to use the unique qualities of some wavelengths to seek out and destroy metastatic tumour cells in lymphatics, veins, and tissues throughout the body at sites remote from the primary tumour.

3. **Development of a True Bloodless Scalpel** - The simultaneous delivery of several wavelengths in the range of the CO_2, argon and Nd:YAG lasers would theoretically offer both the capabilities of cutting and coagulation. The FEL may make it possible to deliver a wavelength which could be used to ablate or excise highly vascular organs such as the liver or some types of vascular tumours with little blood loss.

4. **Reduced Thermal Diffusion** - The ability to select a wider range of powers, wavelengths, and pulse widths may allow for the selective coagulation of blood vessels without thermal damage to surrounding tissues. In addition, the reduced thermal diffusion of some wavelengths may make it possible to drill and cut bone without damaging adjacent live bone.

5. **Tissue Transmission** - the capacity to vary greatly the wavelength and power of the FEL may make it possible to deliver laser energy to tumours or vascular lesions located deep without the body without affecting more superficial and overlying normal tissues and organs.

6. **Intracellular Surgery** - Intracellular surgery on intracellular organelles may be possible with the use of the free electron laser with its wide range of wavelengths, powers, and pulse widths.

7. **Destruction of Infectious Organisms** - It has been hypothesized that infectious organisms including some virus or parasite species can be selectively destroyed by alteration of various subcellular structures such as mitochondria or DNA or RNA. Alternatively, infectious agents may be sensitized by photoactive dyes that react to specific wavelengths of laser light. Thus, the FEL offers some promise for the treatment and/or cure of chronic infections that have resisted traditional chemotherapy.

From the preceding discussion, it is obvious that the free electron laser may make it possible to apply lasers to medicine and gynecology in ways that are more than an extension of current laser technology. Perhaps, the free electron laser may be used to treat gyecologic tumours and infections with a much greater success than is currently possible. One may also anticipate that the development of new wavelengths and powers may create new opportunities for genetic and other intracellular surgery.

CONCLUSION

Although only the future can verify the role of lasers in the treatment of fertility-related disorders, existing clinical experience and investigational work suggest that the lasers will play an ever-increasing role in the future management of reproductive disorders. These developments may make it almost imperative for gynecolgists to become "laser knowledgeable" in order to facilitate their potential use of future lasers. It is important to think beyond the technology and applications of today. With the development of new delivery systems, efficient tunable lasers, and photoactive dyes, lasers may be able to create tissue effects that will greatly enhance our ability to treat human disease.

REFERENCES

1. Bellina JH. Gynecology and the laser. Contemp Obstet Gynecol 1974; 4:24
2. Bellina JH. Reconstructive microsurgery of the fallopian tube with the carbon dioxide laser. Reproduction 1981; 5:1
3. Baggish MS, Chong AP. Carbon dioxide laser surgery of the uterine tube. Obstet Gynecol 1981; 58:111
4. Bruhat M, Mage C, Manhes M. Use of the CO2 laser via laparoscope. In Kaplan I(ed): Laser surgery III, Proceedings of the Third International Society for laser Surgery, Tel Aviv, International Society for Laser Surgery, 1979, 275
5. Tadir Y, Kaplan I, Zuckerman Z, et al. New instrumentation and technique for laparoscopic carbon dioxide laser operations: a preliminary report. Obstet gynecol 1984; 63:582
6. Daniell JF, Brown DH. Carbon dioxide laser laparoscopy: inital experience in experimental animals and humans. Obstet Gynecol 1982; 159:761
7. Daniell JF, Pittaway DE. Use of the CO_2 laser in laparoscopic surgery: initial experience with the second puncture technique. Inferfility 1982; 5:158. Kelly RW, Oberts DK. CO_2 laser laparoscopy: A potential alternative to danazol in the treatment of stage I and II endometriosis. J Reprod Med 1983; 28:638
9. Martin DC. Interval use of the laser laparoscope for endometriosis following danazol therapy. Fertil Steril 1984; 41:735
10. Feste JR. Laser laparoscopy: a new modality. Fertil Steril 1984; 41:745
11. Martin DC. CO_2 laser laparoscopy for the treatment of endometriosis associated with infertility. J Reprod Med 1985; 30:409
12. Nezhat C, Towgey SR, Garrison CP. Surgical treatment of endometriosis via laser laparoscopy. Proceedings of the Annual Meeting of the American Fertility Society. Chicago, Illinois, 1985 (Abstract)
13. Feste JR. CO_2 laser neurectomy for dysmenorrhea. Laser Surg Med 1984; 3:27
14. Keye WR, Dixon J. Photocoagulation of endometriosis by the argon laser through the laparoscope. Obstet Gynecol 1983; 62:383
15. Keye WR, Jr, Hansen LW, Astin M, Poulson AM, Jr. Argon laser therapy of endometriosis: a review of 92 consecutive patients. Fertil Steril 1987; 47:208

16. Lamano JM. Photocoagulation of endometriosis by the argon laser through the laparo-scope. Obstet Gynecol 1983; 62:383
17. Keye WR, Petrucco M, Fowler S. Initial experience with the delivery of the Nd:YAG laser through a sapphire probe. Unpublished data, personal communication.
18. Goldrath M, Fuller T, Segal S. Laser phogocoagulation of endometrium for the treatment of menorrhagia. Am J Obstet Gynecol 1981; 140:14
19. Daniell JF, Meisels S, Miller W, Tosh R. Laparoscopic use of the KTP/532 laser in non-endometriotic pelvic surgery. Colpos and Gynecol 1986; 2:107
20. Daniell JF, Miller W, Tosh R. Initial evaluation of the use the KTP/532 laser in gynecologic laparoscopy Fertil Steril 1986; 46:373

4

Luteal Phase Abnormalities - Diagnosis and Management

DAVID ARCHER

INTRODUCTION

Abnormalities of luteal function are characterized by two distinct clinical entities: a short luteal phase (SLP) and the inadequate or dysfunctional luteal phase (LPD).

The SLP is identified by a luteal interval from LH surge or basal body temperature (BBT) rise to menses of 10 days or less (1). Serum progesterone (P) levels in this condition appear to be normal in terms of mid luteal phase levels and the premenstrual decline. The life span of the corpus luteum based on the following parameters: duration of elevated P, interval from LH surge to menses, and elevation of BBT is approximately 10 days. Whether or not this reflects the formation of a true corpus luteum is debatable. It is possible that luteinization of the follicular apparatus (granulosa and theca cells) has occurred without ovulation taking place. This would be consistent with the luteinized unruptured follicle syndrome.

Conversely luteal phase deficiency or dysfunction (LPD) has a 14 ± 2 day interval based on BBT graphs, and the interval from LH surge to menses (2). Serum P and urinary pregnanediol (PG) levels are significantly less than normal throughout the luteal phase in women with LPD. The endometrial biopsy which reflects the biologic activity of P has been considered to be the sine qua non for diagnosis of LPD. The endometrium is out of phase or lagging behind the expected or anticipated day of the cycle by more than 2 days using the Noyes criteria for histologic dating (3).

INCIDENCE OF LUTEAL PHASE ABNORMALITIES

Both SLP and LPD are associated with infertility and early reproductive (pregnancy) loss (1,2,4). The incidence of SLP has been estimated to occur in anywhere from 10 to 30% of menstrual cycles based on evaluation of BBT graphs in otherwise normal women (1). SLP has also been described following the use of clomiphene citrate (CC) and human menopausal gonadotropin (hMG) administration in both normal women and women with anovulatory infertility (5,6,7,8).

The principal occurrence of SLP is at the time of puberty, when maturation of the hypothalamic-pituitary-gonadal axis occurs (9,10). Both anovulation and SLP occur frequently during the first year post menarche in a significant number of normal women. A comparable increased occurrence of SLP has been documented in female rhesus monkeys during the 1-2 years subsequent to menarche. The SLP in humans has been identified principally by using BBT graphs, but in the rhesus monkey it is based on serum levels of luteinizing hormone (LH), estradiol-17 beta (E2) and P (9,10).

The occurrence of LPD is estimated to be approximately 3-5% of infertile couples (2). The iatrogenic occurrence of LPD may be as high as 30-40% following use of CC and 10-15% in women who have been administered hMG for ovulation induction (5,10).

EXPERIMENTAL INDUCTION OF LUTEAL PHASE DYSFUNCTION

Human: Both CC and hMG administered to stimulate ovulation or initiate multiple follicular development have as a side effect the development of LPD (5,7,11). The exact mechanism that results in LPD following iatrogenic initiation of follicular development is unknown.

Administration of CC to induce ovulation as well as to counteract the estrogen induced inhibition of pituitary gonadotropin secretion has been found to result in both SLP and LPD (6,12). A recent review of LPD indicates that 30-40% of women who receive CC may develop LPD. Currently SLP has only occasionally been documented with CC utilization.

hMG therapy has been used therapeutically in order to treat LPD. Recent experience indicates that 10% of women undergoing hMG administration will have histologic changes compatible with a LPD (8,12). Moreover, the use of hMG in stimulation protocols for in vitro fertilization (IVF) designed to induce multiple follicular development has been associated with a significant occurrence of SLP (7).

Rhesus Monkey: Over the course of investigation into the reproductive physiology of the rhesus monkey, an experimental animal model was developed that was rendered hypo-gonadotropic secondary to lack of endogenous LH-RH (13). This model relied upon electrolytic lesions being placed in the arcuate nuclei of the hypothalamus resulting in the ablation of the neurons that secreted LH-RH. Restoration of pituitary-gonadal function in this animal model was brought about by the exogenous hourly administration of synthetic LH-RH intravenously over several months. A critical evaluation of the data obtained from this model indicates that the initial cycle of follicular development was often accompanied by a less than normal LH surge and a short luteal phase.

Use of the same intermittent LH-RH replacement schedule in prepubertal female rhesus monkeys was also found to initiate ovarian folliculogenesis and ovulation (13). These data indicate that the onset of puberty is secondary to the development of endogenous cyclic LH-RH release. In the initial induced cycle in prepubertal females the ovarian follicular activity has what appears to be a short luteal phase. Continued administration of intermittent LH-RH in both of these experimental situations result in normal ovulatory cycles with a luteal interval of approximately 14 days.

Studies in the luteal phase of the cycle using the above described arcuate nucleus lesioned animals have been performed to determine the role of pituitary LH in supporting the corpus luteum (15). Exogenous LH-RH was administered at hourly intervals until an LH surge was detected. Approximately 3-4 days following the identified LH surge the frequency of the exogenously administered LH-RH was reduced to once every 8 or 24 hours (16).

When LH-RH was infused every 8 hours a normal luteal interval in terms of days from LH surge to menses, and serum P levels was present (16). However, reducing the frequency of LH-RH to one bolus every 24 hours initially maintained serum P levels for 3 days, but ultimately resulted in a fall of serum P levels with the onset of premature menstruation (16). In this experimental situation the finding of a shortened luteal interval was comparable to that seen in the clinically identified SLP.

BIOCHEMICAL CHANGES IN FEMALES WITH A SHORT LUTEAL PHASE

The initial studies that assessed hormonal changes in women with SLP appear to be serendipitous (1). In these women serum follicle stimulating hormone (FSH) was significantly lower than that found in normal women, during comparable times in the follicular phase of the cycle (17). This resulted in an alteration in the FSH/LH ratio. This altered ratio has also been described in rhesus monkeys who were found to have spontaneous SLP (18). Along with the description of a shortened luteal phase in the human was the finding of rather normal serum P levels for 4-6 days following the LH surge. 17 OH-progesterone (17P) was found to be markedly reduced in both the pre and post LH surge interval of the cycle. These findings led to speculation that the altered FSH/LH ratio resulted in a poor stimulation of the granulosa-theca cells of the developing follicle with a subsequent poor or inadequate corpus luteum.

Comparable findings for FSH, FSH:LH ratio and serum P levels have been reported in the female rhesus monkey in both spontaneously occurring SLP and in an experimentally induced SLP following the exogenous administration of charcoal absorbed ovine follicular fluid (18).

PUBERTY AND THE OCCURRENCE OF SHORT LUTEAL PHASES

As previously described initial administration of exogenous LH-RH to female rhesus monkeys results in a short luteal phase in the first ovarian stimulatory cycle, with progression to a normal luteal interval. Comparable findings have been reported in both human and rhesus females at the time of puberty (9,10,19). There is a high incidence of luteal phase defects, principally SLP, in human females during the first 1-2 years past menarche (1). This luteal dysfunction disappears to be replaced by a normal luteal interval and normal menstrual cycles.

A detailed hormonal investigation performed in post pubertal female rhesus monkeys indicated a high frequency of SLP (9). In this study FSH, LH, P and E2 patterns were evaluated. The initial post menarchal ovarian cycles, characterized by SLP, were ultimately replaced by normal menstrual function and intervals. However, repetitive SLP cycles existed for up to 2 years.

SHORT LUTEAL PHASE IN THE HUMAN

Based on the above clinical and experimental evidence it is hypothesized that SLP in the human could be due to a reduction in the quantitative amount of pituitary LH released during the luteal phase. Studies are currently being undertaken to investigate LH pulse frequency and amplitude during the luteal phase of the cycle. To date complete studies exist in only 2 women with SLP compared to 2 normal women, and these studies are inconclusive. However, daily blood samples obtained throughout the menstrual cycle indicate that women with SLP have a prolonged follicular phase, a quantitatively reduced LH surge, and a significantly lower P level at the time of the LH surge. These data are initial observations and require confirmation. They are of interest since the occurrence of SLP in our experience with hMG for follicular recruitment has occurred more often when follicular maturation is delayed.

THERAPY FOR LUTEAL PHASE ABNORMALITIES

As can be seen from the preceding description, the precise pathophysiology of luteal phase abnormalities is unknown. Present therapy for both SLP and LPD is empirical and the success rate in terms of successful pregnancy outcome is not known.

Initial management of spontaneously occurring SLP and LPD is CC. Dosage schedules should be the same as that used for anovulation beginning with 50 mg of CC per day from days 5-9 following menstruation. After three cycles of treatment CC is arbitrarily increased to 100 mg per day for 5 days. BBT monitoring for evidence of a short luteal interval (a thermogenic shift of < 10 days) should be performed. During the third cycle of CC 100 mg per day an appropriately timed endometrial biopsy should be obtained.

If there is evidence of a persistent SLP or LPD, then hMG therapy should be administered. At present the author sees no advantage in the use of CC plus human chorionic gonadotropin (hCG) treatment. Standard hMG protocols should be used with appropriate monitoring of serum or urinary E2 levels, and ultrasound imaging of the developing follicles. During the hMG treatment cycle if there has been no clinical evidence of SLP, a timed endometrial biopsy should be obtained in the third treatment cycle.

Evidence for either LPD and/or SLP during hMG treatment is now becoming more prevalent. A consensus approach to treatment is not available, but the administration of exogenous intermittent LH-RH throughout the entire menstrual cycle is being used at this time. Use of pure FSH (Metrodin) rather than hMG does not appear to offer any advantage, nor does multiple small doses of hCG administered throughout the luteal phase.

Appropriate medical management of both SLP, and LPD await further investigation into the pathophysiology of these clinical entities. It is anticipated that the increased information will help in selecting appropriate therapy for these individuals.

REFERENCES

1. Strott CA, Cargille CM, Ross GT, Lipsett MB. The short luteal phase. J Clin Endocrinol Metab 1970; 30:246
2. Jones GS. The luteal phase defect. Fertil Steril 1976; 27:351
3. Noyes RW, Hertig AT, Rock J. Dating the endometrial biopsy. Fertil Steril 1950; 1:3
4. Kusuda M, Nakamura G, Matsukuma K, Kurano A. Corpus luteum insufficiency as a cause of ovulatory failure. Acta Obstet Gynecol Scand 1983; 62:199
5. Cook CL, Schroeder JA, Yussman MA, Sanfilippo JS. Induction of luteal phase defect with clomiphene citrate. Amer J Obstet Gynecol 1984; 149:613
6. Vaitukaitis JL, Bermudez JA, Cargille CM, Lipsett MB, Ross GT. New evidence for an anti-estrogenic action of clomiphene citrate in women. J Clin Endocrinol Metab 1971; 32:503
7. Jones GS. The role of luteal support in a programme for in vitro fertilization. In Implantation of the Human Embryo, eds Edwards RH, Purdy J,Steptoe PC, Academic Press, London, United Kingdom, 1985; p285
8. Olson JL, Rebar RW, Schreiber JR, Vaitukaitus JL. Shortened luteal phase after ovulation induction with human menopausal gonadotropin and human chorionic gonadotropin. Fertil Steril 1983; 39:284
9. Foster DL. Luteinizing hormone and progesterone secretion during sexual maturation of the rhesus monkey : Short luteal phase during the initial menstrual cycles. Biol Reprod 1977; 17:584
10. Ryan KD. Maturation of the hypothalamic-pituitary axis regulating gonadotropin secretion in the primate. Sem Reprod Endocrinol 1986; 4:3
11. Kubik CJ, Albert JL, Tobon H, Archer DF. Incidence of luteal phase defect during ovulation induction with human menopausal gonadotropin (hMG). Abstract 37 presented at the 1986 meeting of The American Fertility Society, Toronto, Canada

12. Kubik CJ. Luteal phase dysfunction following ovulation induction. Sem Reprod Endocrinol 1986; 4:293

13. Knobil E, Plant TM. The neuroendocrine control of gonadotropin secretion in the female rhesus monkey. In Frontiers in Neuroendocrinology, Eds Ganong WF, Martin L, New York, Raven Press, 1978 p249

14. Wildt L, Marshall G, Knobil E. Experimental induction of puberty in the infantile female rhesus monkey. Science 1980; 207:1373

15. Hutchison JS, Zeleznik AJ. The corpus luteum of the primate menstrual cycle is capable of recovering from a transient withdrawal of pituitary gonadotropin support. Endocrinology 1985; 117:1043

16. Hutchison JS, Zeleznik AJ. Effects of varying gonadotropin pulse frequency on corpus luteum function and lifespan during the menstrual cycle of rhesus monkeys. Endocrinology 1986; 119:1964

17. Sherman BM, Korenman SG. Measurement of plasma LH, FSH, estradiol and progesterone in disorders of the human menstrual cycle. The short luteal phase. J Clin Endocrinol Metab 1974; 3889

18. Wilks JW, Hodgen GD, Ross GF. Luteal phase defects in the rhesus monkey: The significance of serum FSH:LH ratios J Clin Endocrinol Metab 1976; 43:1261

19. Winter JSD, Faiman C. The development of cyclic pituitary-gonadal function in adolescent females. J Clin Endocrinol Metab 1973; 37:714

5

The Gonadotropin-Resistant Ovary

ROGER D KEMPERS

Reproduced in part in Postgraduate Obstetrics and Gynecology
Volume 7, no. 6, 1987

INTRODUCTION

In this day of great interest in in-vitro fertilization and tubal microsurgery for women who have no other options to conceive, it is important to keep in mind those occasional patients who, although they appear to be menopausal, retain the capacity to conceive. Patients with the gonadotropin-resistant ovary syndrome represent a fascinating subset of women in the spectrum of those who develop premature ovarian failure because these women have ovaries which still contain oocytes.

Premature ovarian failure is characterized by the cessation of ovarian function after puberty and before the age of 40. This occurs in about one percent of women. Patients with premature ovarian failure have no demonstrable genetic abnormality and grow normally during adolescence. Premature ovarian failure represents one extreme in the spectrum of disorders constituting premature gonadal failure. Premature gonadal failure includes patients such as those with gonadal dysgenesis and true hermaphroditism whose failure occurred prenatally. Chromosome analysis allows proper delineation of these disorders. Those associated with a karyotype containing a Y chromosome have a defect in testicular differentiation. Those containing X chromosome monosomy or other abnormalities of the X chromosome have defects in ovarian differentiation. Patients with postnatal premature gonadal failure have 46 XX chromosome analysis, implying that the ovaries have undergone differentiation and once functioned normally. A recent review of the experience at the Mayo Clinic of 182 patients seen with gonadal failure between 1970 and 1980 revealed that 22, or 12 percent, were due to defects in testicular differentiation; 78, or 43 percent, were due to defects in ovarian differentiation; and 82, or 45 percent, were due to failure in postnatal maturation (1).

Table 1 is a classification modified from Lim et al of this third category -- those with postnatal premature ovarian failure (2). The vast majority are patients with premature follicular depletion. There are, however, occasional patients with postnatal premature gonadal failure who have the gonadotropin-resistant ovary syndrome. Patients with premature follicular depletion may exhibit either primary or secondary amenorrhea. As shown in Table 1, the etiology may be variable, but the majority are of idiopathic etiology. In approximately 10 percent of women with premature ovarian failure, there is a positive family history of a similar disorder which suggests the possibility of inheritance or a genetic etiology (2). The suggestion has been made that there may be either an autosomal-dominant or X-linked pattern in these patients. As noted previously, of the 182 patients with gonadal failure in the Mayo Clinic study, 82 were examples of postnatal maturation defect. Twelve of these patients had primary amenorrhea. Sixty-six patients had secondary amenorrhea without remaining follicles, and 4 had secondary amenorrhea with remaining follicles. Two of those patients were examples of the gonadotropin-resistant ovary syndrome, one was due to autoimmune disease, and one was due to intraovarian hemorrhage.

Table 1 Postnatal premature ovarian failure

I. **Premature follicular depletion**

  A. Autoimmune disease
  B. Familial
  C. Iatrogenic
  D. Infectious
  E. Secondary to systemic disease
  F. Idiopathic

II. **Unresponsive retained follicles**

  A. Gonadotropin-resistant ovary syndrome
  B. Autoimmune disease
  C. Idiopathic

DIAGNOSTIC CRITERIA

In 1969, Jones described 3 women who had the combination of premature ovarian failure, hypergonadotropic amenorrhea, and apparently normal ovarian follicular apparatus (3). Neither increasing the endogenous gonadotropins with clomiphene citrate nor the administration of massive doses of exogenous gonadotropins, with human menopausal gonadotropins, induced a significant increase in follicular estrogen production or ovulation. She sugested that these ovarian follicles were resistant to gonadotropin stimulation. The condition became known as the gonadotropin-resistant ovary syndrome. A recent review of the literature by Maxson and Wentz revealed that only 14 cases have been reported which satisfy the criteria for diagnosis (4). Multiple other cases have been reported but lack sufficient data to permit inclusion in a substantive study of this condition. Criteria essential for diagnosis are: (1) primary or secondary amenorrhea, (2) secondary sexual development, (3) intact uterus and vagina, (4) numerous primordial follicles on ovarian biopsy, (5) 46, XX karyotype, (6) elevated gonadotropin concentrations, (7) resistance to exogenous gonadotropins, and (8) absence of concomitant autoimmune disease. This is a report summarizing two additional cases studied at the Mayo Clinic in the past 10 years.

CASE REPORTS

In the first case, menarche occurred at age 10. From age 17 to 20, she took oral contraceptives; and upon discontinuing these, she was amenorrheic. Withdrawal menses did not occur with intramuscular progesterone. At age 23, at another institution, she was diagnosed as having adrenogenital syndrome. She was treated with prednisone for several months, but remained amenorrheic. A withdrawal menses was then produced with oral medroxy-progesterone, and the following month she conceived. Following delivery of a normal-term infant, she developed oligomenorrhea. Scant menses occurred at varying intervals of up to 6 months, and she experienced hot flashes.

When studied at age 29, the general and pelvic examinations were satisfactory. There was no evidence of hirsutism. Normal endocrinologic studies included urinary 17 ketosteroids and ketogenic steroids, pregnanetriol, plasma total testosterone, serum total and free thyroxine, basal prolactin, and fasting blood sugar. The serum LH was elevated to 5 times normal, the serum FSH was elevated to 7 times normal, and the serum total estrogen was reduced to 3 ng/dl. The blood karyotype analysis was 46 XX. Degenerative bone changes were noted in the thoracic and lumbar spines. At laparotomy, both ovaries were 5 x 2 x 2cm, atrophic, and nodular. For diagnostic purposes, wedge biopsies were removed from each, and these revealed the presence of primordial follicles. There was a corpora albicans in one ovary. No corpora lutea were identified. There was atrophic endometrium on curettage. The diagnosis of gonadotropin-resistant ovary syndrome was thus confirmed. She was placed on cyclic oral contraceptives and supplemental calcium carbonate. Several years later, still not interested in further childbearing, she reported having regular withdrawal bleeding on the oral contraceptive therapy and was free of hot flashes.

In the second case, menarche occurred at age 14; and thereafter she had irregular menstrual periods. She conceived and delivered a term infant at age 20. She then took oral contraceptives until age 26. When these were stopped, she remained amenorrheic. Withdrawal bleeding was then produced with conjugated estrogens and medroxyprogesterone in cyclic fashion over a period of 8 months. On discontinuing this medication, she again became amenorrheic.

When studied at age 31, the general and pelvic examinations were satisfactory. There was no evidence of hirsutism. Normal endocrinologic studies obtained at that time included serum basal prolactin, total serum thyroxine, and plasma total testosterone. The serum FSH was elevated to 2 times the upper limits of normal. The serum LH was elevated to 5 times normal. The serum total estrogen was decreased to less than 3 ng/dl. The blood karyotype analysis was 46 XX. A diagnostic laparoscopic procedure was performed.

This revealed the right ovary to be 4cm in diameter and the left ovary 2.5cm in diameter. A biopsy of the right ovary revealed a few primordial follicles present within a fibrous cortical ovarian stroma. There were several hyalinizing corpora albicans identified. The diagnosis of gonadotropin-resistant ovary syndrome was made, and replacement hormonal therapy was recommended.

ANALYSIS OF DATA

An analysis of the findings from these two cases and the 14 cases previously reported was made. Six, or approximately 40 percent, had primary amenorrhea; and 10, or approximately 60 percent, had secondary amenorrhea. In the latter group, the average age of cessation of menses was 22.4 years with a range of 13 to 31 years. The average time span from menarche to menopause was 9.2 years. The character of the menstrual cycle in those patients with secondary amenorrhea was variable. Menarche occurred at an average age of 13.2 years. Secondary sexual development of both breast and pubic hair was reported as normal in all 16 cases. However, increased amount of sexual hair was reported in three patients who were mildly hirsute. The occurrence of normal breast development in patients wiht secondary amenorrhea is expected. The source of estrogen in patients with primary amenorrhea is either the ovary itself or peripheral aromatization of ovarian and adrenal androgens. The gonadotropin-resistant ovary syndrome may be an acquired or incomplete phenomenon. The production of small amounts of ovarian estrogen from developing follicles or theca and stroma at the beginning of puberty could stimulate the initial development of secondary sexual characteristics. All patients had a normally developing uterus and vagina except for one patient with a unicornous uterus.

The ovarian morphology is noteworthy. A requirement of the gonadotropin-resistant ovary syndrome is the demonstration of numerous primordial follicles on ovarian biopsy. In this series, only one patient did not have this histologic picture of ovarian biopsy. The biopsy was performed laparoscopically. The superficial fragment of ovarian cortex contained no primordial follicles or corpora albicantia. This patient was included as a case of gonadotropin resistance because human menopausal gonadotropin did produce withdrawal bleeding in one cycle. Subsequently, she did conceive. The inadequate biopsy failed to detect the presence of follicles. To establish the diagnosis of this syndrome, an adequate ovarian biopsy should be obtained. This can be best accomplished by laparotomy and ovarian wedge resection.

Any woman with this syndrome who is less than 30 years of age should have karyotype analysis to rule out the presence of Y chromosomal material and its associated 20 precent risk of ovarian neoplasms such as gonado-blastoma or dysgerminoma. Those patients with sex chromosomal mosaicism and a chromosomal complement which includes a 45 X cell line can thus be identified. Occasionally, patients with 45 X karyotype, with or without mosaicism, will demonstrate spontaneous initiation of menses, ovulation, and even pregnancy prior to the onset of premature ovarian failure. A normal 46 XX karyotype must be present to establish the diagnosis of gonadotropin-resistant syndrome.

The gross and histologic description of the ovaries are of interest. The ovaries were described grossly as small or normal. The surfaces of these gonads were unstimulated and showed no evidence of corpora lutea or developing follicles. The biopsies from our 2 cases showed the presence of numerous primordial follicles. Histologically all ovaries in the 16 cases reviewed except the ones with the inadequate biopsy, had numerous primordial follicles. In several biopsies, a few follicles in the early antral stage of development as well as follicles in various stages of atresia were demonstrated. None of these specimens exhibited a corpus luteum, but 6 of the 16 biopsies, including 2 cases in this report, did have corpora albicantia, indicating that luteinization, and presumably ovulation, had once occurred. None had leukocyte infiltration, which accompanies autoimmune ovarian failure. In patients with established ovarian failure, there is an associated elevation in the gonadotropin concentration. In these cases, the diminished levels of estradiol and ovarian peptides failed to exert a negative feedback suppression on the hypothalamic/pituitary axis. In this series, all patients had concentrations of gonadotropin which were in the menopausal range. These patients are characterized by a resistance to stimulation by exogenous gonadotropins. While the process of ovarian follicular development from the primordial follicle to the early antral stage is independent of gonadotropins, small amounts appear to facilitate this process. Much higher doses of FSH are required to stimulate granulosa cell mitosis, estradiol production, increase in FSH receptors, and further stimulation of follicular growth from the early antral to the graafian preovulatory follicle.

No patients with documented autoimmune disease are included in this series. As stated, none demonstrated leukocyte infiltration of the ovary on biopsy or clinical evidence of autoimmune disease. Nevertheless, the gonadotropin-resistant ovary syndrome may ultimately prove to be a manifestation of autoantibodies to FSH receptors or gonadotropins.

PATHOGENESIS

A review of theories of the pathogenesis of the gonadotropin-resistant ovary has been outlined by Maxsom and Wentz (4). A number of possibilities exist. Since these patients all exhibit normal secondary sexual characteristics, even when associated with primary amenorrhea, it is evident that this disorder is acquired after the estrogenic stimulus to thelarche, which accompanies early puberty. Many of these patients have secondary amenorrhea., indicating that the defect can be acquired or incomplete. Theories regarding the pathogenesis of this syndrome include (1) abnormal FSH molecule, (2) FSH receptor defect, (3) autoimmune phenomena, (4) absence or nonresponsiveness of target cells and (5) 46, XX gonadal dysgenesis.

Abnormal FSH

Although inactivity of FSH itself could produce the gonadotropin-resistant ovary syndrome, there is no evidence to support this likelihood. Normal bioactivity of FSH has been demonstrated in patients with this syndrome. Furthermore, attempts to stimulate ovarian response with exogenous gonadotropins up to 10 times that required to induce ovulation in patients with hypopituitarism has generally been unsuccessful in stimulating an ovarian response in these patients. Other investigators have failed to detect abnormal LH or FSH by gel filtration in patients with this syndrome.

FSH Receptor Defect

The implication of resistance by the ovary to superphysiologic concentrations of apparently normal endogenous or exogenous gonadotropins is that there may be a defect at the level of the target cell itself. FSH receptor function could be absent either due to interference with normal FSH function, a congenital pausity or receptors, or defective function within the receptors themselves following normal gonadotropin function. The presence of normal secondary sexual characteristics in these patients, even in those with primary amenorrhea, suggests that there has been some estrogen production by those few follicles that had some normally functioning receptors.

Defective function of the gonadotropin receptors themselves seems possible. The binding of peptide hormones to cell-membrane bound receptors stimulates the adenylate/cyclase system. The possibility exists that insufficient cAMP could account for resistance to gonadotropin stimulation.

Autoimmune Disease

Autoimmune disorders may be caused or associated with immune response, be it cellular or hormonal, against the body's own antigens. One cause of premature ovarian failure has been shown to be the autoimmune phenomenon. Support for this concept has been the known association of autoimmune phenomena and premature failure in a number of cases, the demonstration of circulating antibodies to be the ovary in sera of women with this disorder, and the association of lymphocytic infiltration found in ovaries of patients with this condition. The blocking of the effectiveness of FSH and LH by antibodies to gonadotropins or to the receptors themselves may evolve at anytime. Autoimmune ovarian failure has been associated with the syndrome of polyglandular failure. In these cases, it has been associated with adrenal insufficiency, Hashimoto's thyroiditis, Graves' disease, pernicious anemia, Addison's disease in as many as 10 to 20 percent of cases of this disease, and in myasthenia gravis where there have been antibodies directed against acetylcholine as well as gonadotropin receptors. Circulating anti-ovarian antibodies have been demonstrated by radioimmunofluorescence and ligand-binding. The ovarian antigen that binds to antibody in premature ovarian failure is the subject of continuing investigation. In these ovaries, lymphocytic and plasma cell infiltration can be found around primordial follicles. It is believed that the autoimunity results from a defect in immunoregulation rather than in the effector cells.

Target Cell Dysfunction

Theoretically, there may be another defect in the target cell beyond the binding of gonadotropins and stimulation of cAMP production. Investigation of the integrity of the target cell response to adenylate/cyclase in patients with a syndrome of gonadotropin insensitivity is needed.

46 XX Gonadal Dysgenesis

The possibility exists that one step in the evolution of the gonadotropin-resistant ovary is the exhausting of primordial follicles in patients with pure 46 XX gonadal dysgenesis. It has been suggested that in some instances these ovaries evolve with time from small hypoplastic gonads to true streak ovaries rather than to the atrophic ovary characteristic of the menopause. In 2 patients with hypogonadotropic secondary amenorrhea, unilateral streak ovary, and contralateral hypoplastic ovary, with follicles documented on biopsy, laparotomy several years later revealed the presence of bilateral streak ovaries with no evidence of follicles (4). Thus the syndrome of gonadotropin resistance in a few patients may represent one point in the evolution of follicular exhaustion associated with 46 XX gonadal dysgenesis. To confirm this observation, it would be necessary to perform repeated ovarian biopsies in patients with gonadotropin-resistant syndrome.

THERAPY

Pregnancies have been reported in women with a diagnosis of gonado-tropin-resistant syndrome. These pregnancies have occurred spontaneously or have followed cyclic estrogen and progesterone treatment or the administration of menopausal gonadotropins (4). However, only a limited number of these reports of successful therapy are sufficiently documented to be convincing. No patients with primary amenorrhea and the gonadotropin resistant syndrome, regardless of the various therapeutic modalities, have conceived. In these cases, since congenital absence of some aspect of the FSH receptor is the most likely causative factor, there is no specific therapy one can recommend for infertility. In patients with secondary infertility, where the diagnosis most likely rests in some acquired interference with binding at the receptor, trials of therapy with different modalities are reasonable. Shanghold and Hammond in 1977 reported a patient who conceived during a 5-month course of cyclic estrogen and progesterone therapy (5). This patient received conjugated estrogen 2.5 mg daily for 21 days each month with supplemental medroxyprovera. Another well-documented case by Lim and associates was reported in 1984 (6). Estrogens and progesterones were given cyclically for 2 months with inadequate suppression of serum FSH and LH concentrations. When the therapy was discontinued, a rebound increase of the serum gonadotropin concentrations was observed. Ethinyl estradiol was prescribed for 2 1/2 months and serum LH and FSH concentrations were suppresed significantly. After cessation of the therapy, regular menstrual periods resumed. Initially, the cycles were anovulatory but subsequently became ovulatory. Nearly two years later, she conceived. It was postulated that since FSH was suppressed over a period of time the cells were no longer exposed to the antigen, and this allowed them to recover. The developing follicles then developed normal FSH receptors and were no longer insensitive to gonadotropins.

When the association of autoimmune phenomena with premature ovarian failure is established by the demonstration of circulating antibodies to the ovary and the presence of lymphocytic infiltrate in the ovarian biopsy, steroid immunosuppressive therapy may be tried. The return of menstrual function has been documented in a number of cases. However, no cases of subsequent pregnancy have been reported. We reported on one such patient in whom this diagnosis was established. She was maintained on prednisone therapy and the return of menstrual function was documented. Ultimately, she developed polyglandular failure and returned to an amenorrheic state (7).

Because these young women with premature ovarian failure are at high risk for developing osteoporosis, it is imperative that they be maintained on estrogen and progesterone therapy as well as supplemental calcium. Progesterone should be given for 10 to 14 days each month to reduce cytoplasmic receptors for estrogen and reduce the risk of endometrial carcinoma.

Patients with no ovarian function have another important option for pregnancy. The methodology for nonsurgical recovery and transfer of in vivo fertilized donated ovum is now established. The first delivery of a neonate to an agonadal woman following transfer of an in vitro fertilized ovum from another infertile patient was described in 1984; also that year, the first delivery of a neonate following nonsurgical donor-ovum transfer was reported (8). More recently, pregnancy and delivery in two women with ovarian failure was reported following nonsurgical transfer of in vivo fertilized uterine ova (9). In these latter two patients, the mothers were first treated with oral conjugated estrogens and intramuscular progesterone for one cycle. Steroid supplementation was continued through the twentieth week of gestation. In the first patient, the blastocyst was recovered from the donor on the first insemination cycle and, in the second, following the third insemination cycle.

SUMMARY

Two new cases of gonadotropin-resistant ovary syndrome have been described and discussed in combination with the 14 other well-documented cases recently reviewed in the literature. Although examples of the gonadotropin-resistant ovary syndrome are infrequent, they are a significant cause of premature ovarian failure. The pathogenesis of this condition is not clearly understood. It is likely that the defect lies in either a congenital absence of FSH receptors or inhibition of binding of FSH to the receptor. This may be due either to autoimmune disease or to destruction of the FSH recptors by some other etiology. The diagnosis of this syndrome is established by the finding of elevated gonadotropin concentratrions and numerous primordial follicles on ovarian biopsy. Patients with gonadotropin-resistant ovary syndrome retain their pregnancy potential. Cyclic estrogen and progesterones will suppress FSH, and newly developing follicles, in some cases, regain gonadotropin sensitivity. In patients with autoimmune phenomena, the use of immuno-suppression with glucocorticoids seems reasonable. Although menstrual periods occasionally resume, to date, no pregnancies have been reported.

The possibility of the gonadotropin-resistant ovary syndrome should be considered in the differential diagnosis of all women with premature menopause. These patients should be followed for the possibility of later development of autoimmune phenomena and should be maintained on estrogen, progesterone, and calcium supplements.

REFERENCES

1. Coulam CB. Premature gonadal failure. Fertil Steril 1982; 38:645-655
2. Friedman CR, Barrows H, Kim MH. Hypergonadotropic hypogonadism. Am J Obstet Gynecol 1983; 145:360-372
3. Jones GS, de Moraes-Ruebsen M. A new syndrome of amenorrhea in association with hypergonadotropism and apparently normal ovarian follicular apparatus. Am J Obstet Gynecol 1969; 104:597-600
4. Maxsom WS, Wentz AC. The gonadotropin-resistant ovary syndrome. Seminars in Reproductive Endocrinology 1983; 1:147-160
5. Shangold MM, Turksoy RN, Bashford RA, Hammond CB. Pregnancy following the "insensitive ovary syndrome". Fertil Steril 1977; 28:1179-1181
6. Lim HT, Meinders AE, DeHann LD, Bronkhorst FD. Anovulation presumably due to gonadotropin-resistant ovary syndrome. Eur J Obstet Gynecol Reprod Biol 1984; 16:327
7. Coulam CB, Kempers RD, Randal RV. Premature ovarian failure: evidence for the autoimmune mechanism. Fertil Steril 1981; 36:238-240
8. Lutjen P, Traunson A, Leeton J et al. The establishment and maintenance of pregnancy using in vitro fertilization and embryo donation in a patient with primary ovarian failure. Nature 1984; 307:174-175
9. Formigli L, Formigli G. Pregnancy and delivery in two women with ovarian failure following nonsurgical transfer of in vivo fertilized ovum. JAMA 1986; 256:1442

6

Laser Treatment in Female Reproductive Surgery

JAMES F DANIELL

Lasers have been used in many fields of medicine for years, but there is not enough understanding among gynecologists of the various lasers that can be clinically used today in gynecology. This chapter will review the physics of lasers in general, specifically the carbon dioxide laser. A general overview of the clinical uses now possible, both endoscopically and at open laparotomy in areas of female reproductive surgery, will be briefly summarized.

PHYSICS OF LASERS

Laser is an acronym for light amplification by stimulated emission of radiation. A laser produces and amplifies visible and near visible light creating intense, coherent electromagnetic energy which can be reflected off mirrors to bring it to a target site. A lens can focus the energy to small spot sizes and concentrate the energy to high power densities. Past the focal point, the beam defocuses and creates large spot sizes with low power densities.

Laser Components

A laser generally consists of a pumping system, an optical cavity, a lasing media and electronic controlling panel. The pumping system excites the atoms to higher energy states.

The optical cavity has parallel mirrors at either side producing continuous reflection. One mirror is partially silvered which allows the photons to pass out of the system and down posts carrying the beam to a target. This cavity is similar to any resonator cavity which allows amplification of waves.

The lasing media may be a solid state media such as a crystal of Ruby or Neodymium: Yttrium Aluminium Garnet, a gas such as helium, neon or carbon dioxide, a complex organic dye, or semiconductor such as gallium arsenide diode.

The electronic controlling system controls the pumping and exit of the laser. The wattage increases the number of atoms which are pumped to higher states. The pulsing technique opens and closes a shutter to allow exit of the continuous laser. These pulses can be directly controlled by the length of time the foot is on the pedal or can be set for finite pulses or varying lengths. Superpulse modes have been designed to produce the cooling advantages of a pulsed mode but the action of a continuous mode. This cooling decreases the thermal spread and decreases the peripheral tissue fibrosis. The use of pulses is one of two prime techniques for controlling tissue reaction.

Power Density

The prime control of tissue effect is by controlling the power density. Concepts and knowledge of power density and its control is essential for proper use of the laser. The power density is defined as:

$$PD = \frac{Power}{r^2}$$

As can be seen from this formula, the power density is directly related to the power output measured in wattage and inversely related to the square of the radius of the spot size. Smaller spot sizes increase power density more effectively than changing the power. A change in spot diameter from 2mm to 0.2mm increases the power density 100-fold (Table 1).

Table 1 The tissue effect of various power densities of the CO_2 laser

Power density Watts/cm^2 *	Action
0 to 5	Warming
5 to 300	Superficial contraction/coagulation
300 to 1,200	Excisional vaporization
1,200 to 15,000	Incisional vaporization
15,000 to 100,000	Rapid incision

* Watts/cm^2 are calculated

Tissue Effect

The laser beam may be transmitted, reflected, absorbed or scattered. Transmission allows passage of the laser to its target site. Reflection off mirrors helps guide and change the direction of the laser. Absorption of the laser beam produces tissue response. Scatter is a redirecting of the laser beam as it impacts on the tissue.

TYPES OF SURGICAL LASERS

The three main types of lasers used in surgery are Carbon Dioxide, Argon and neodymium: Yttrium Aluminium Garnet (Nd:YAG). Developmental work involves Krypton, Tunable Dye, Excimer and Potassium Titanyl Phosphate (KTP) Crystal lasers.

Carbon Dioxide Laser

The Carbon Dioxide laser is most commonly used for vaporization for either ablation or excision. The residual tissue has a remnant coagulation zone which generally varies from 100 microns to 500 microns. The depth of this zone is directly related to the time used to make the incision and the power density. Rapid incisions at high power densities can hold the zone to 100 microns. Lower power denisty and slower incisions can increase the zone to 500 microns.

Ablation implies complete vaporization of the target tissue into a smoke plume. Excision implies vaporization of an underlying zone to lift the lesion off so that it can be sent for pathological examination.

The CO_2 laser has an infrared wave length of 10.6 microns. The beam is absorbed by nonreflective solids and liquids, especially water containing tissue. Water containing tissues absorb the laser power in the first 100 microns. Depth of coagulation past this is generally related to the heat of vaporization.

This absorption is not dependent upon the colour of tissue and has minimal scattering. The degree of hemostasis is directly related to the depth of coagulation. A 500 micron coagulation zone seals off the larger vessels better than the 100 micron coagulation zone. Thus the higher power densities and rapid incisions produce less coagulation and less hemostasis while leaving less necrotic tissue behind.

Although the CO_2 laser is predominantly a vaporizing laser, it is possible to use this for coagulation of surface peritoneum. This is most useful if performing cuff salpingostomies. With this technique, the laser can be used with a very low power density of around 50 watts per square centimeter to coagulate and contract the serosal surfaces of the hydrosalpinx. This turns the hydrosalpinx back in a cuff fashion.

In addition, the CO_2 laser can be directed along polished mirror systems. These lasers also deliver sufficient power for intra-abdominal surgery from very compact units operating off ordinary electrical outlets.

The radiation of the CO_2 laser is nonmutagenic as the effect is due to the absorption and conversion of radiant heat to energy. This is similar to the

74

radiant energy that can be absorbed when sitting in front of a fireplace. This is different than the ionizing radiation of x-rays and gamma rays. Although the CO_2 laser itself is nonmutagenic, the plume has the same mutagenic potential as cigarette smoke.

LASER SAFETY

The topic of laser safety is more complex than can be covered adequately in a single chapter. A manual such as 'Laser Safety in Medicine and Surgery' should be read and understood.

The laser with its immense power and no touch technique has more potential for damage than the knives surgeons have used since childhood and than cautery which has caused bowel and ureteral burns. Education in laser use should come from 'hands-on' courses and practice in the surgeon's own operating room using surgical specimens or other objects. Hand-held and microscopic practice techniques are easy enough to design. Models for laparoscopic techniques can be as complex as specifically built metal boxes or as easily available as taping two plastic dishpans together and cutting holes in them for access with laparoscopes and for suction.

In general the following should be observed:

- Limit access to room and laser key
- Have a qualified laser technician run the laser
- Use correct safety eyeglasses for the specific wave length of the laser to be used
- Have adequate suction to remove the carbon plume from the operating field as this plume has the same mutagenicity as cigarette smoke
- Avoid contact with the inside power generating circuits which store up to 15,000 volts
- Avoid flammable cleaning solutions and anesthetic gases
- Use flame retardant surgical drapes
- Use general anesthesia when appropriate to decrease the chance of unexpected motion of the patient
- Flood the pelvis with solutions or cover other areas with moistened packs to avoid inadvertent injury with the laser
- Use backstops such as quartz rods, pyrex rods, etched metal rods, soaked sponges or water solutions to limit the penetration of the laser
- Use front surfaced polished metal or front surfaced glass mirrors to reflect the beam. Back surfaced glass mirrors will fracture and front surfaced mirrors can be vaporized

- Monitor the EKG at laparoscopy when the extended operating time increases the chance of CO_2 absorption
- Be prepared to use cautery as the laser does not provide absolute hemostasis
- Protect from hypothermia due to heat loss with the multiple washings used to remove carbonized material from the pelvis at laparotomy or laparoscopy
- When possible remove all carbonized particles as these remain in the pelvis for extended periods of time and may produce a foreign body giant cell reaction

CLINICAL USES FOR LASERS

Surgical lasers have now been used in reproductive surgery hysteroscopically (1,2), laparoscopically (3-14) and at open laparotomy (15-25). Clinically, most work has been done with the CO_2 laser because that laser has been commercially available for the longest period of time and has other applications in gynecology. The CO_2 laser has been used at open abdominal surgery, both articulated to the operating microscope with a special micromanipulator or using a handpiece which attaches directly to the laser. There are advantages and disadvantages of both methods of use of the laser. Some of these differences are listed in Table 2.

At laparotomy, the CO_2 laser has been used for almost all types of reconstructive pelvic surgery (Table 3). Although many of the postulated benefits at laparotomy are controversial, most authors agree that in certain

Table 2 Comparison of methods of using the CO_2 laser at open abdominal surgery

	Microscope	Hand-held scalpel
Requires extra hardware	Yes	No
Easy to use deep in pelvis	Yes	No
Mirror use possible	Yes	Yes
Easy to vary spot size	No	Yes
Magnified tissue view is possible	Yes	Yes, with loupes
Good light visibility	Yes	Yes, with fiberoptic headlight
Fine control of beam with micromanipulator	Yes	No
Simple assembly	No	Yes

76

circumstances the laser decreases operating time, decreases blood loss, increases the ease of operation and decreases operator strain. The effect on adhesion reformation, pregnancy rates, occurrence of pain and re-operation rate is still under study. The studies that are available are still too small for comparison of specific techniques, but appear to be equivalent to results found with microsurgical techniques (15, 16, 19, 20, 25).

Table 3 Operations that have been performed with the intra-abdominal CO_2 laser both hand-held and with microsurgical attachments

1. Excision of endometriosis
2. Lysis of adhesions
3. Cuff salpingostomies
4. Cornual re-implantation
5. Tubal transection in preparation for anastomosis
6. Fimbrioplasties
7. Metroplasties
8. Myomectomies
9. Salpingostomies for excision of ectopic pregnancies
10. Ovarian wedge resection
11. Uterosacral ligament vaporization

Mage (18) and Tulandi (21) have reported on cuff salpingostomies using the microsurgical laser. Mage reported 9 term pregnancies in 38 patients followed for 21 months. In addition, he reported 4 abortions and 3 ectopic pregnancies. Tulandi reported 3 term pregnancies in 11 patients followed for 10 months.

Diamond(22) followed a mixed group of patients undergoing laser surgery (both hand-held and microsurgery) for both adhesive disease and endometriosis. There were 38 term pregnancies in 106 patients. There were also 2 abortions and 2 ectopics. Chong(23) reported on 6 months of follow-up in a group of patients with endometriosis. Fourteen of 23 patients with mild endometriosis had become pregnant. Eleven of 13 with moderate endometriosis and 3 of 8 with severe endometriosis had also become pregnant.

Kelly(19) reported 3 pregnancies in 28 patients undergoing salpingostomies followed for 12 months. Two of these progressed to term and 1 was a tubal pregnancy. He also reported 4 term pregnancies and 1 abortion in 21 patients undergoing adhesiolysis. Eight patients out of 12 undergoing tubal reversal had term pregnancies. He further reported 2 term pregnancies and 1 abortion in 8 patients treated for pathologic occlusion.

McLaughlin(24) performed myomectomies on 18 patients and metroplasties on 3 patients. Five of the myomectomy patients had become pregnant at 12 months of follow-up. Four had either delivered or were progressing uneventfully. One ectopic pregnancy had occurred. In addition, he performed metroplasties on 3 patients. There have been no pregnancies in this group.

LASER LAPAROSCOPY

The obvious advantages of using the CO_2 laser laparoscopically are that if the procedure can be accomplished, major surgery and its undesired expenses and sequella can be avoided. Those physicians who have become competent in the field of laser laparoscopy have uniformly found that they are able to extend their ability to do more difficult procedures, thereby avoiding laparotomy in certain situations. Clinical data is beginning to accumulate that uniformly appears to support the early claims that the CO_2 laser beam can be used under laparoscopic control with accuracy, with safety and with good clinical results. This new modality has been successful for treatment of endometrosis for infertility and/or pain, and treatment of other conditions such as distal tubal obstruction and temporary relief of anovulation associated with polycystic ovarian disease. The various types of surgical procedures that are possible with the CO_2 laser laparoscope are listed in Table 4. As can be seen, almost every type of operative laparoscopic procedure that has been previously attempted has been accomplished using CO_2 laser technology.

Table 4 Operations that have been performed with the CO_2 laser laparoscope

1. Vaporization of endometriosis
2. Terminal neosalpingostomy for hydrosalpinx
3. Uterosacral ligament ablation
4. Pelvic adhesiolysis
5. Vaporization of small uterine fibroids
6. Ovarian cystotomy
7. Ablation of hydatid cysts
8. Vaporization of ovarian fibromas
9. Multiple cystotomy in polycystic ovarian disease
10. Linear salpingostomy for ectopic pregnancy

The present endoscopic delivery systems for the CO_2 laser are somewhat cumbersome and technically difficult because of the necessity for firing the CO_2 beam through air or a gas medium. Researchers have been investigating flexible CO_2 delivery systems, but at present, none are commercially available. Another potential method of use for the CO_2 laser consists of delivering the beam through a long, rigid probe that may be used under fluids or used through an endoscope, such as a hysteroscope or a laparoscope. This concept, if possible, would allow delivery of the beam in a manner similar to that presently available with fibers for other lasers.

At present, many commercial companies are marketing equipment for CO_2 laser laparoscopy. Equipment available includes second puncture delivery systems and delivery systems for using the laser beam through the operating channel of a modified laparoscope. The present state-of-the-art equipment allows the interested laparoscopist who becomes familiar with the CO_2 laser to effectively use this technology. The only instrument that is required is a surgical CO_2 laser with an articulated arm and a helium neon beam that is bright enough to be visualized laparoscopically.

CREDENTIALING

Hospitals have a significant problem deciding who should be privileged (credentialed) to perform which procedures (delineation). For many hospitals, the procedure for doing this is recommended by the departmental chairman or by a small group without objective or specific guidelines to determine competence for the specific procedure. In recent years, hospitals have been held liable under a theory of corporate negligence when physicians are allowed to perform procedures before specific competence has been demonstrated. More than ever, hospitals have a responsibility and liability as to determining who should be allowed to provide which services(26, 27).

Medical staff bylaws of most hospitals place the burden upon the physician to demonstrate that he or she has met certain prerequisites before performing specific procedurs. Residencies and fellowships have generally provided the necessary prerequisite education and experience for gynecologic surgery. Although there are some residencies and fellowships that do meet the necesary guidelines, laser surgery, particularly intra-abdominal laser surgery, is felt by many to be in an area where the general training provided in residencies and fellowships is not adequate.

THE FUTURE OF LASERS FOR INFERTILITY SURGERY

Many new lasers are being developed and evaluated for potential use in gynecology. Specifically, the argon and the potassium titanyl phosphate (KTP) laser seem promising for operative laparoscopy. Both of these lasers can be delivered by flexible 600 micron fibers for treatment of endometriosis or adhesions laparoscpically. Early reports on clinical use of these new lasers seem promising with investigators reporting similar results to the CO_2 laser with much easier delivery techniques(28, 29).

Hysteroscopic laser surgery for infertility problems is in its infancy. CO_2 laser prototypes for hysteroscopy have proved unworkable. The argon, the KTP and the Nd:YAG lasers are all being evaluated in clinical trials as hysteroscopic treatment for uterine septi, submucosal fibroids and intra-uterine adhesions. Preliminary reports are encouraging for treating all these problems but further work is needed before any firm conclusion can be drawn.

Theoretically, the free electron laser which can be tuned to any desired specific wavelength may have future uses in infertility, but it has yet to be evaluated by gynecologists. The Excimer laser which delivers pulsed energy at 308 nanometers in one billionth of a second bursts and which cuts with no heat transfer to tissue may also be useful in infertility surgery in future.

CONCLUSIONS

Lasers are here to stay in gynecologic infertility surgery, both open and endoscopic. Meaningful data is just beginning to appear in the literature to show that laparoscopic laser treatment is safe and effective therapy for both endometriosis and adhesive disease.

Further critical evaluation of both open abdominal and hysterosopic laser surgery continues. All thoughtful gynecologists interested in female repro-ductive surgery should carefully evaluate the potential for using surgical lasers and closely follow the activities in this exciting area of gynecology.

GLOSSARY

Continuous wave   Continuous output of the laser beam

Pulsed Laser   A true pulsed laser stores its energy to be released in one instant

Laser "Pulse"   Pulses of a continuous wave laser can be used to decrease the thermal spread

Superpulse   Electronic pulsing of a continuous wave laser designed to increase thermal spread and decrease tissue damage

Photovaporization	Ablation of tissue in the absorption zone by flash vaporization
Photocoagulation	Coagulation of the tissue in the field without removing the tissue
CO_2	Carbon dioxide
Nd:YAG	Neodymium: Yttrium Aluminium Garnet
TEM	Transverse electromagnetic mode
Spot Size	The calculated theoretical spot size of the laser beam at a plane in space. The minimum spot size is calculated at the focal length of the laser.
Power Density	The calculated, theoretical concentration of power when the laser impacts on tissue
HeNe	Helium Neon laser used as aiming beam with the CO_2 or Nd:YAG laser

SUGGESTED READING

"Laser Safety in Surgery and Medicine" Fourth Edition, Ed. J. Rockwell, Cincinnati: Rockwell Associates, 1983. Distributed by Lase, Inc., 8150 Corporate Park Drive, Suite 222, Cincinnati, Ohio 45242

"Perioperative Laser Nursing" Ed. C. J. Mackety, Thorofare, NJ: Slack Inc., 1984

"Laser Surgery in Gynecology and Obstetrics" Ed. W. R. Keye, Boston: G. K. Hall, 1985

"Basic and Advanced Laser Surgery" Ed. M.S. Baggish, Norwalk: Appleton-Century-Crofts, 1985

REFERENCES

1. Goldrath M, Fuller T, Segal S. Laser photovaporization of endometrium for the treatment of menorrhagia. Am J Obstet Gynecol 1981; 140:14-19
2. Tadir Y, Raif J, Dagan J, Kaplan I, Zuckerman Z, Ovadia J. Hysteroscope for CO_2 Laser Application. Lasers Surg Med 1984; 4:153-156
3. Daniell JF, Brown DH. Carbon dioxide laser laparoscopy: initial experience in experimental animals and humans. Obstet Gynecol 1982; 59:761
4. Daniell JF, Pittaway DE. Use of the CO_2 laser in laparoscopic surgery: initial experience with the second puncture technique. Infertility 1982; 5:15

5. Tadir Y, Kaplan I, Zuckerman Z, Edelstein T, Ovadia J. New instrumentation and technique for laparoscopic carbon dioxide laser operations: a preliminary report. Obstet Gynecol 1984; 63:582
6. Kelly RW, Roberts DK. Laser laparoscopy: a potential alternative to danazol in the treatment of stage I and II endometriosis. J Reprod Med 1983; 28:638
7. Martin DC. Interval use of the laser laparoscope for endometriosis following danazol therapy. Fertil Steril 1984; 41:74S
8. Feste JR. Laser laparoscopy: a new modality. Fertil Steril 1984; 41:74S
9. Daniell JF, Herbert CM. Laparoscopic salpingostomy utilizing the CO_2 laser. Fertil Steril 1984; 41:558
10. Bruhat M, Mage C, Manhes M. Use of the CO_2 laser via laparoscopy. In Laser Surgery III, Proceedings of the Third Internation- al Society for Laser Surgery, Edited by I Kaplan Tel Aviv, International Society for Laser Surgery, 1979, p 275
11. Keye WR, Matson GA, Dixson J. The use of the argon laser in the treatment of experimental endometriosis. Fertil Steril 1983; 39:26
12. Keye WR, Dixson J. Photocoagulation of endometriosis by the argon laser through the laparoscope. Obstet Gynecol 1983; 62:383
13. Lamano JM. Photocoagulation of early pelvic endometriosis by the Nd:YAG Laser through the laparoscope. J Reprod Med 1985; 30:86
14. Daniell JF. Polycystic ovaries treated by laparoscopic CO_2 laser vaporization. Obstet Gynecol (in press)
15. Daniell JF. The role of lasers in infertility surgery. Fertil Steril 1984; 42:815
16. Diamond MP, Feste J, Daniell JF, McLaughlin D, Martin DC. Pelvic adhesions at early second look laparoscopy following carbon dioxide laser surgical procedures. Infertility 1984; 7:39-44
17. Daniell JF, Diamond MP, Feste J, McLaughlin D, Martin DC. Clinical results of terminal salpingostomy using the CO_2 laser: Report of the Intra-abdominal laser study group. Fertil Steril (in press)
18. Mage G, Bruhat MA. Pregnancy following salpingostomy: comparison between CO_2 laser and electrosurgery procedures. Fertil Steril 1983; 40:472
19. Kelly RW, Roberts DK. Experience with the carbon dioxide laser in gynecologic microsurgery. Am J Obstet Gynecol 1983; 146:585
20. Bellina JF. Microsurgery of the fallopian tube with the carbon dioxide laser: analysis of 230 cases with a two year follow up. Laser Surg Med 1983; 3:255
21. Tulandi T, Farag R, McJunes RA, Gelfand MM, Wright CV, Vilos GA. Reconstructive surgery of hydrosalpinx with and without the carbon dioxide laser. Fertil Steril 1984; 42:839
22. Diamond MP, Daniell JF, Martin DC, et al. Tubal patency and pelvic adhesions at early second look laparoscopy following intra-abdominal use of the carbon dioxide laser: initial report of the intra-abdominal laser study group. Fertil Steril 1984; 42:717
23. Chong AP, Baggish MS. Management of pelvic endometriosis by means of intra-abdominal carbon dioxide laser. Fertil Steril 1984; 41:14
24. McLaughlin DS. Micro-laser myomectomy technique to enhance reproductive potential: a preliminary report. Lasers Surg Med 1982; 2:107
25. Daniell JF. The CO_2 laser in infertility surgery. J Reprod Med 1983; 28:265
26. Dorsey JH, Baker CH. Credentialling of the gynecologic laser surgeon. Colp Gyn Laser 1984; 1:79
27. Dorsey JH, Baggish MS. Initialing a CO_2 laser program. In "Basic and Advanced Laser Surgery in Gynecology", Baggish MS (ed.). Appleton-Century-Crofts, Norwalk, 1985, pp 373-381
28. Daniell JF. Laparoscopic Use of the KTP/532 Laser in Nonendometriotic Pelvic Surgery. Colp Gyn Surg 1986; 2:107
29. Daniell JF. Initial evaluation of the use of the potassium titanyl- phosphate (KTP/532) laser in gynecologic laparoscopy. Fertil Steril 1986; 46:000

7

Management of Hyperandrogenisation in Women with Polycystic Ovarian Disease

F H M TSAKOK

K H CHAN

C S A NG

Disorder of androgen secretion is a much commoner condition in the Asian female than has been heretofore realised. It presents itself in a variety of clinical manifestations. Since it causes chronic anovulation with potential serious consequences, a greater incidence of infertility, endometrial carcinoma and breast carcinoma, the physician must understand the situation and undertake therapeutic measures to avoid these sequelae.

NORMAL ANDROGEN PRODUCTION

The production rate of testosterone in the normal female is 0.2 to 0.3 mg/day (1). Approximately 50% of testosterone arises from the peripheral conversion of androstenedione while the adrenal gland and ovary contribute approximately equal amounts to the circulating levels of testosterone (2). Production of dehydroepiandrosterone sulphate arises exclusively from the adrenal glands. Together with the other ketosteroids, dehydroepiandrosterone and androstenedione are quantitatively the most abundant androgens (3) in the normal female. Androgenicity is dependent upon the unbound fraction of testosterone of which 80% is bound to the betaglobulin, sex hormone binding globulin and another 19% bound to albumin (4).

Ovarian androgen production occurs principally in the theca and the ovarian interstitial tissue and is under the control of pituitary gonadotrophins (5). Progesterone competes with testosterone for 5 alpha reduction and so may influence the effects of testosterone (6). Peripheral metabolism of androgens to the active dihydrotestosterone is by 5 alpha reduction but androgens such as androstenedione can be converted to oestrone in the peripheral fatty tissue (8).

HYPERANDROGENIC STATE

The most sensitive marker of increased androgen production is hirsutism but in Asian women it has been shown that this is an uncommon presentation (9). It has been shown that hyperandrogenism may not be associated with hirsutism because of decreased 5 alpha reductase activity in the skin (10). The hyperandrogenic state is more commonly expressed as menstrual irregularity, acne or increased oiliness of the skin.

Extreme androgenic effects of virilisation such as male hair pattern, clitoromegaly, deepening of the voice, increased muscle mass and general male body habitus are rare. If masculinisation develops over several months the most common causes are drugs (the 19 nortestosterones, danazol and anabolic agents). Although androgen producing tumours, adult onset adrenal hyperplasia and incomplete testicular feminisation and mosaics are very rare, they have to be excluded as causes.

The usual source of androgen excess secretion is from the ovaries but may not be exclusively so. In Lobo's series (10) only 50% of patients had raised serum testosterone concentrations whilst the levels of dehydroepiandrosterone sulphate were as often raised. Enlarged polycystic ovaries are not pathognomonic either. Nevertheless in increased androgen secretion the majority of patients have cystic ovaries.

ANDROGEN STATE IN CHINESE WOMEN

In an analysis of a series of 107 infertile Asian women of Chinese ethnic origin seen in 1983 (Kandang Kerbau Hospital, Singapore) inappropriate gonadotrophin secretion of LH:FSH ratio more than 2 occurred in 23.4%. Four percent had raised levels of dehydroepiandrosterone sulphate (DHEAS) whilst serum testosterone level was raised in 12%.

Hirsutism was not a complaint in any patient whilst abnormal menstrual bleeding occurred in all. Ovaries visualised at laparoscopy were smooth and sclerocystic in all cases but only 4% were enlarged.

The incidence of hirsutism in these anovulatory infertile women of Chinese descent is low and is similiar to the findings of Aono and co-workers (9) in Japanese women.

RESULT OF INDUCTION OVULATION

When infertility is a problem induction of ovulation with antioestrogens is the treatment of choice. Of the 25 women with raised LH:FSH ratio and anovulation tamoxifen citrate was used in 12 cases. As in most studies (12) there seems no therapeutic advantage when using tamoxifen in clomiphene nonresponders. In the present series 78% who use clomiphene and 66.6% who use tamoxifen showed a biphasic temperature pattern demonstrating that both the negative and positive feedback mechanisms are intact (13). The ovulation rate is representative of similar studies (14) but only 16.6% (3 patients) conceived with antioestrogen treatment alone. This may be explained by the high incidence of low progesterone levels obtained 7 days after presumptive ovulation (<10ng/ml) in 49%. The incidence of luteal phase insufficiency has been noticed to be high in women with polycystic ovaries treated with clomiphene (15).

Clomiphene plus human chorionic gonadotropins (hCG) has been used in those who fail to ovulate with antioestrogens alone. There was no success in this series. This sceptism about whether the addition of hCG is of any use in clomiphene nonresponders has been expressed before (16).

In the two patients with hyperprolactinaemia, treatment was applied with bromocriptine. One patient who conceived had a spontaneous abortion at 9 weeks.

Four of the clomiphene non-responders, who were also hyperandrogenic, were given corticosteroids (prednisolone 7.5mg o.n.). Ovulatory menses occurred in three patients and one became pregnant. Glucocorticoids suppress adrenal androgen production (17) but has been reported to have an effect on the ovary (18).

Of those who had not conceived with oral treatment parenteral medication with human menopausal gonadotropin can be used. One patient conceived on treatment with pergonal but two out of the three who had treatment suffered from mild to moderate hyperstimulation. In Wang and Gemzell's series (19) 22% had hyperstimultation including some with severe degree requiring hospitaliation showing that women with polycystic ovarian disease are at higher risk of hyperstimulation.

In fact, the pregnancy rate of HMG treatment in polycystic ovarian disease has been disappointingly low and the incidence of pregnancy wastage high 75% (20). The high serum LH in polycystic ovarian disease causes premature luteinisation (21) which may be enhanced by the LH content of HMG (Human Menopausal Gonadotrophin). For the above reason treatment with pure follicle stimulating hormone (FSH) has the advantage in lowering the side effects and increasing the ovulation rate in women with high endogenous LH levels (22).

In a further series of 7 patients treated over 15 cycles using pure FSH (metrodin) (23), the pregnancy rate was 71% (5 out of 7) with 3 hyperstimulated cycles, 2 moderate and 1 requiring hospitalisation. In that study we used low-dose FSH given subcutaneously by a pulsatile infusion pump. Each pulse was regulated at a 90 minute interval starting with an initial dose of 8 units per pulse increasing or decreasing 2 units every three or four days depending on the number of follicles developing and their rate of growth. When the mean diameter of the leading follicle was 18mm as assessed by ultrasound and the endometrium was judged to be preovulatory 10,000 units of hCG was given followed by another 5000 units 7 days later.

All the cycles were completed and were ovulatory (86.6%). There was one with four follicles and another with two follicles. The others were single follicles. The mean amount of FSH given per day was 146 iu/day.

Pregnancy occurred in 5 out of 7 patients. There were two singleton pregnancies and one twin pregnancy with viable births. There was one 10 week abortion and a premature delivery of a triplet pregnancy at twenty seven weeks resulting in neonatal deaths. Finally there were two chemical pregnancies. This low dose pulsed FSH regimen has had an encouraging success rate of ovulation and pregnancy as has been noticed by Franks and co-workers (24).

Pulsatile LHRH has been used for inducing ovulation in cystic ovaries (23, 25). As has been noticed by others (26) we have found the treatment successful in achieving ovulation with the advantage of unifollicular ovulation. In our series of 5 women treated with pulsatile LHRH through 9 cycles, there were 7 ovulatory cycles. The pregnancy rate was poor with one chemical pregnancy and another clinical pregnancy which aborted at 12 weeks (40%) gestation. There were, however, no cases of hyperstimulation.

CONTROL OF POLYCYSTIC OVARIAN DISEASE

When fertility is not a problem, cystic ovarian disease is still of concern to the physician since the characteristic polycystic ovary emerges when a state of anovulation persists for any length of time.

In cystic ovaries new follicular growth is continuously stimulated but not to the point of full maturation and ovulation. Multiple follicular cysts less than 10mm diameter are formed which are surrounded by hyperplastic theca cells often luteinised in response to high levels of LH. As various follicles undergo atresia, they are immediately replaced by new follicles of similar limited growth potential. The number of growing and atretic follicles are much increased.

With this excessive follicular maturation and atresia, the ovary is rapidly depleted of primordial follicles and therefore decreasing fertility potential further. The stroma also becomes hyperplastic. There is an increase in production of androgen in the form of androstenedione which can be converted peripherally to oestrone and testosterone. This in turn causes a decrease in sex hormone binding globulin with an increase in free oestradiol. Evidence indicates that the elevated LH, due to hypersensitivity of the pituitary is attributed to the increased oestrogen levels. Chronic anovulation is perpetuated and uninterrupted oestrogen stimulation may give rise to an increased risk of endometrial and breast cancer (27). In this series of infertile patients, one developed endometrial carcinoma and her reproductive career had to be abandoned.

In another group of 38 women complaining of menstrual abnormalities seen in 1983, with inappropriate gonadotropin ratio and no imminent fertility problems, 55% had irregular heavy bleeding whilst 20% had prolonged episodes of amenorrhoea. Only one patient actually complained of hirsutism whilst 74% had troublesome acne and visible facial hair. Only 39% were obese. Testosterone levels were high in 60% and dehydroepiandrosterone sulphate (DHEAS) high in 5% of patients.

The abnormal bleeding in these patients was controlled by giving cyproterone 50 mg daily for 2 months followed by a combination oral contraceptive pill containing 2 mg of cyproterone acetate (Diane).

Acne and hirsutism were well controlled. Periods became regularised. The treatment was stopped after two years. The levels of androgen and LH were normalised. In 8 patients who had wanted a pregnancy after treatment, 6 have conceived showing that spontaneous ovulation and fertility occurs in a substantial number of patients.

The plan is to resume treatment after two years should symptoms and the hyperandrogenic state recur to prevent the sequelae of prolonged oestrogen stimulation and conserve fertility.

REFERENCES

1. Speroff L. Anovulation in Clinical Gynaecologic Endocrinology and Infertility, eds Speroff L, Glass R, Kase N, William & Wilkins.
2. Bardin, Lipsett M. Testosterone and Androstenedione blood production rates in normal women and women with idiopathic hirsutism and polycystic ovaries. J Clin Invest 1967; 46: 891.
3. Osborn R H, Yannone M E. Plasma androgens in normal and andorgenic female, a review. Obstetrical and Gynaecological Survey 1971; 26:195
4. Anderson D C. Sex-hormone binding globulin. Clin Endocrin (Oxf) 1974; 3:69-73
5. Tsang B K, Armstrong D T, Whitfield J F. Steroid Biosynthesis by isolated human ovarian follicular cells invitro. Clin Endocrin and Metab 1980; 54:1407
6. Morris D V. Hirsutism. Clin Obstet Gynaecol 1985: 649-674
7. Toscano V, Petrangeli E, Admamo M V et al. 1981 Simultaneous determination of 5 alpha reduced metabolites of testosterone in human plasma J Steroid Biochem 1981; 14:574
8. Edman C D and MacDonald P C. Effect of obesity on conversion of plasma androstenedione to estrone in ovulatory and non-ovulatory young women Am J Obstet Gynecol 1978; 130:456-461
9. Aono T, Miyazaki M, Miyake A, et al. Responses of serum gonadotrophins to LH - releasing hormone and oestrogens in Japanese women with polycystic ovaries. Acta Endocrinol 1977; 85:840
10. Lobo RA 1985. Disturbances of Androgen Secretion and Metabolism in Polycystic Ovarian Syndrome. in Clin Obstet Gynaecol 1985; 663-647
11. Goldzieher J W, Green J A. The polycystic ovary I Clinical and Histologic Features. J Clin Endocrinol Metab 1962; 22:325-338
12. Klopper A, Hall M. New Synthetic agent for the induction of ovulation Preliminary trials in women. Br Med J 1971; 152-154
13. Jacob H S, Hull M G R, Murray M A F, Franks S. Therapy orientated diagnosis of secondary amenorrhoea. Horm Res 1975; 6:268-287
14. Garcia J E, Seegar Jones G E, Wentz A C. The use of clomiphene citrate. Fert Steril 1977; 30:617-630
15. Yen S S C, Vela P, Ryan K J. Effect of clomiphene citrate in polycystic ovarian syndrom : Relationship between serum gonadotrophin and corpus luteum function J Clin Endocrinol Metab 1970; 31:7-13
16. Yen S S C 1978. Chronic anovulation due to inappropriate feedback system. In Yen S S C & Jaffe (eds) Reproductive Endocrinology 1978 p 297-323, Philadelphia : W B Saunders

17. Perloff W H Smith K D, Stein Berger E. Effect of prednisolone on female infertility. Int J of Fert 1965; 10:31-40
18. Kircher M A Zucker R, Jespersen D et al. Idiopathic hirsutism - an ovarian abnormality. New Engl J Med 1976; 294:637-640.
19. Wang C F, Gemzell C. The use of human gonadotrophins for the induction of ovulation in women with polycystic ovary disease. Fert Steril 1980; 33:479-486
20. Lunenfeld B, Inster V. Diagnosis and Treatment of Functional Infertility Grosse Verlay Berlin 1978; 61-89
21. Coutts J R T, Hamilton M P R, Black W P, Daxton M, Fleming R. A New Successful Treatment for Infertile Women with Polycystic Ovarian Syndrome Abstracts of VII International Congress of Endocrinology 1984
22. Kamrava M M, Seibel M M, Berger M, Thompson I, Taymor M L. Reversal of persistent anovulation in polycystic ovarian disease by administration of chronic low-dose follicle stimulating hormone. Fert Steril 1982; 37:520-523
23. Tsakok F H M, Ng C S A, Chew S C. Pulsatile urofollitropin (Pure FSH) and luteinising hormone releasing hormone (LHRH) for induction of polycystic ovarian disease (PCOD). Proceedings of the Third Congress of Endocrinology Asean Federation of Endocrine Societies p F57, 1985
24. Franks S, Mason H, Polson D, Saldahna M B Y. Induction of ovulation with low dose pulsatile FSH in women with polycystic ovary syndrome J Endocrinol 1985; 104 (Supplement) :605
25. Jacobs H S, Porter R N, Abdul Wahid N A, Honour H W, Craft I. Gonadotrophic determination of the intrafollicular environment. In Programme of the III World Congress of IVF Melbourne, 1985.
26. Burger C W, Van Kessel, Schoemaker V, et al. Induction of ovulation by prolonged pulsatile administration of luteinising hormone releasing hormone (LHRH) in patients with clomiphene resistant polycystic ovary like disease. Acta Endocrinol 1983; 104:357-364
27. Cowan L D, Gordis L, Tonascia Y A, Jones G S. Breast cancer incidence in women with a history of progesterone deficiency. Am J Epidemiol 1981; 114:209

8

Transvaginal Sonographically Controlled Oocyte Recovery for IVF

WILFRIED FEICHTINGER

Ultrasound guided aspiration of oocytes for IVF began with the trans-abdominal and transvesical approach pioneered by Susan Lenz and her colleagues in Scandinavia (1, 2). The needle guided technique holds a number of advantages and we have developed it for use through the transvaginal route. Essentially, there is a transducer with a needle guide which can guide the direction and depth of penetration of the needle. The needle is marked on the ultrasound monitor with a dotted line and if the dotted line is aimed to pass through the maximum diameter of the ovarian follicle then the needle will be aimed to enter that particular follicle (1, 2, 3).

If the ovaries are located in the pouch of Douglas then the transvesical approach is not very effective since the distance separating the ovary from the transducer is very long. In 1985, a transvaginal probe was developed in collaboration with the Kretztechnik company. Work in this area has evolved over the past decade, for instance, Kratochwil in Vienna started experimental work with transvaginal scanning 20 years ago! However, because ultrasound was not well developed at that stage the idea was abandoned.

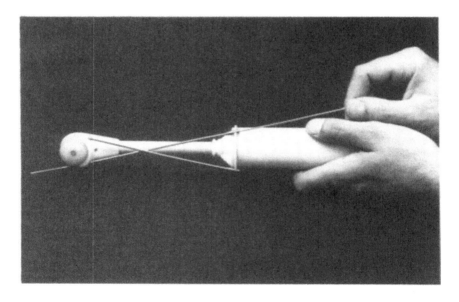

Figure 1 Transvaginal probe

The probe that is currently used in our department (Figure 1) is a rotating front-looking sector scanner probe which can be used at 5 and 7.5 MHz frequency. The probe is quite small and at its maximum diameter it is only about 3cm wide. The probe is long and this allows it to be inserted into the lateral fornices reducing the distance between the probe and the ovaries (Figure 2). A sector scanner gives better pictures than a linear array but most of the sector scanners which are presently on the market have only an approximately 90-degree field of vision. In comparison, the probe used in our department has a 240 degree field of vision and is therefore called a panoramic scanner. The scanner can be applied in the longitudinal, transverse and oblique views and is very useful not only in in vitro fertilisation but also for general pelvic scanning.

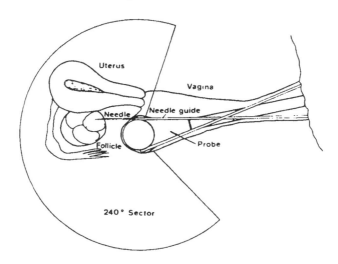

Figure 2 Placement of probe

When the probe is used for puncturing procedures 2 metal tubings set at 15 degrees towards the scanner axis are attached to it and serve as needle guides and prevent the needle from injuring the vaginal walls (Figure 2).

The procedure of puncturing itself can be manually guided with a short single lumen needle of 1.4mm outer diameter or by an automated puncture device which is spring loaded (4).

The depth of puncture can be controlled by adjusting the depth limiting screw of the device. The needle of the puncturing device is long with a narrow dead space and is therefore outfitted with a double lumen. This allows aspiration of the oocyte through the first channel and fluid to be flushed through the second. There is, therefore, less chance of losing the egg.

Figure 3 shows an ovary with 3 large follicles. There are two puncture lines on the monitor which correspond to the two channels. There are centimetre markings on the monitor which are equivalent to the actual depth of

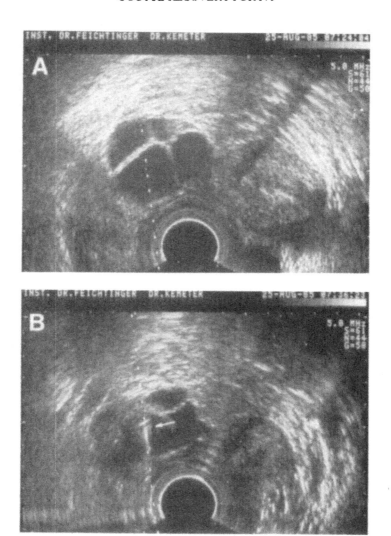

Figure 3 Transvaginal follicle puncture. A: Three preovulatory follicles in the left ovary. The dotted guideline passes through one of these follicles (the first to be aspirated). B: The needle has been inserted with the needle tip (arrow) inside the follicle, and aspiration has begun.

penetration by the automated puncturing device. Once a follicle is punctured the follicle will collapse. If no egg is recovered in the initial aspirate then the follicle should be flushed and re-aspirated. When flushing begins bubbles will be obtained and part of the view of the needle lost. If this happens, the needle should be held tight.

RESULTS OF ULTRASOUND-GUIDED FOLLICLE ASPIRATION

The results of 649 ultrasound-guided follicle aspirations (both transvesical and transvaginal approaches) compared to 279 laparoscopic oocyte recoveries are shown in Table 1. Laparoscopy was performed both at the University Clinic (Vienna) and at a private outpatient center (Institute of Reproductive Endocrinology and In Vitro Fertilization, Vienna). The oocyte recovery rate of both groups was 83.8% (522 oocytes from 623 follicles of more than 2ml contents). With ultrasound guidance, the appropriate figures were 1,623 oocytes from 1,891 follicles, i.e. 85.8% (5). The clinical pregnancy rate was highest in the group with the ultrasound-guided oocyte retrieval (22%); however, the "take-home baby rate" was similiar (14.9%) to that obtained at the private outpatient center where laparoscopy was used (16%). This was due to the lower number of abortions in the latter group.

Table 1 Results of ultrasound-guided follicle aspirations compared with laparoscopic oocyte recovery

	Univ. Clinic	Private, outpatient treatment	
	1981/82 Laparoscopy	1982/83 Laparoscopy	1983-Aug 86 USP
Patients	148	62	376
Treated cycles	204	75	649
Embryo replacements	119	50	469
Clinical pregnancies	20 (13.5%)	9 (14.5%)	83 (22%)
Abortions	5	0	20
Ectopic pregnancies	2	0	5
Born children	14 (9.5%) (1 x twins)	10 (16%) (1 x twins)	50 (5 x twins) ⎫ (14.9%)
Children on the way	-	-	16 ⎭ (1 x triplets 1 x twins)

After ultrasound guided follicle aspiration there were 20 abortions and 5 ectopic pregnancies. Sixty-six children were born giving a baby take home rate of almost 15%.

There was no statistical difference between laparoscopic and ultrasound guidance when the pregnancy rates were analyzed according to the number of embryos replaced in each group (5). Comparison of transabdominal (transvesical) follicle aspiration and the transvaginal aspiration technique is shown in Table 2 and the results were almost the same in both groups. Oocyte recovery was successful in 94.6% of transabdominal follicle aspirations and in 97.5% of transvaginal follicle aspirations (i.e., at least one oocyte was recovered per patient). The pregnancy rate was slightly higher after transvaginal oocyte recovery (13.3% per puncture) versus the transabdominal approach (12.4%). The normal pregnancy rate (8.6% versus 9.2%) was not significantly different in the 2 groups.

Table 2 Comparison of transabdominal and transvaginal techniques

	Foll. aspiration by transabd. (transves.) ultrasound guidance	Foll. aspiration with transvag. probe + punct. - device
No. of attempted oocyte recoveries	371	278
No. of successful oocyte recoveries	351 (94.6%)	271 (97.5%)
No. of follicles (> 2 ml)	1568	1372
No. of oocytes	1345 (85.8%)	1180 (86%)
Av. no. of ooc. per oocyte recovery	3.6	4.2
No. of fertilized oocytes	796 (59.2%)	641 (54.3%)
No. of embryo replacements	252 (68%)	217 (78%)
Clinical pregnancies	46 (12.4%/PCT 18%/ER)	37 (13.3%/PCT 17%/ER)
Abortions	8	12
Ectopic pregnancies	4	1
Normal pregn. + deliveries (Baby take home rate)	34 (9.2%/PCT 13.5%/ER)	24 (8.6%/PCT 11%/ER)

COMPLICATIONS OF THE DIFFERENT METHODS OF EGG RECOVERY (Table 3)

Compared to laparoscopic oocyte recovery the incidence of severe complications using ultrasound-guided follicle aspiration was low. Out of a total of 203 laparoscopies, three laparotomies were necessary: two because of bowel-perforation (one with a trocar, one with coagulating forceps), and one because of postoperative bleeding from the ovary. Many patients suffered

Table 3 Complications of different methods of follicle puncture

	Foll. asp. by laparoscopy	Foll. asp. by transabd. (transves.) ultrasound	Foll. asp. with transvag. probe + punct. - device
No. of treatments	204	371	278
Puncture of bowel	2	7	3
Puncture of blood vesssel	0	6	6
Punct. of uterus or uterine fibroma	0	7	6
Haematuria	0	14	0
Severe postoperative pain	> 10% (gas!)	3	0
Laparotomies necessary after foll. puncture	3 (2**,1***)	(1)	0
Infections in vitro	14 (6.8%) (Husb.)	27 (7.2%) (Husb.)	14 (5%) (Husb.)
Infections in vivo	0	2 (cystitis)	(1?) *

* pelvic inflammation 3 months after puncture
** severe bowel injuries
*** intraabd. bleeding from ovary

from postoperative pain due to the residual gaseous distension of the abdomen. It can therefore be seen that the conventional method using laparoscopy for oocyte recovery may result in a number of problems, especially if there are significant adhesions in the pelvis. In comparison bowel puncture occurred in 7 of 371 cases using the transabdominal approach and in 3 of 278 transvaginal ultrasound-guided punctures. There were no complications from these bowel punctures, and in all cases with suspected or confirmed puncture of bowel, prophylactic antibiotic treatment was given. The iliac vein was mistakenly punctured for a follicle on six occasions but this resulted in no complications. A repeat scan showed no intraabdominal hemorrhage in any of these patients. Out of 371 cases of transvesical puncture, 14 patients had moderate hematuria lasting at least 1 day, but there were no episodes of severe hematuria. Two patients developed cystitis after puncture, one of whom had a prior history of chronic urinary tract infection. Three patients had severe postoperative pain after transabdominal (transvesical) puncture. One of these patients had an exploratory laparotomy that revealed no pathological finding. To date, this complication has not occurred after any of the transvaginal punctures. One patient was treated for pelvic inflammatory disease 3 months after transvaginal follicle aspiration but it is unclear if there was a causal association between the 2 events. Infections did not occur more frequently after transvaginal puncture than in the two other groups (5), and most, if not all, of these cases were probably caused by infection of the semen.

CONCLUSIONS

The vaginal approach for follicle aspiration has the advantage of a shorter puncture route. With other techniques, the bladder has to be entered, and the puncture route is longer. With transvaginal sonography, the bladder is empty and is not along the pathway of the follicle-aspirating needle. Owing to the elastic nature of the vagina, the tip of the ultrasound probe can be brought into close proximity to the ovary. If loops of bowel are in the path to be transversed by the needle, they can be displaced by manipulating the probe. As indicated previously, even if a loop of bowel is inadvertently punctured by the fine needle, it does not appear to result in significant complications. Using the transvaginal technique, even ovaries located high up in the pelvis can be reached. In comparison with transvesical oocyte retrieval, the transvaginal approach is less painful, easier to perform, and there are no bladder problems following the procedure. There is no need for general anesthesia or even sedative medication. In summary we feel that transvaginal sonographically controlled oocyte recovery should replace both laparoscopy as well as other ultrasound guided follicle aspiration techniques for IVF.

USE OF TRANSVAGINAL APPROACH FOR INDICATIONS OTHER THAN IVF

1. In Gynaecology

Numerous other gynecologic diagnoses are possible with the new vaginal sector scanner probe: monitoring of follicle numbers and size using serial pelvic ultrasound examinations during a stimulation cycle, clear visualization of the uterus and endometrium, excellent imaging of the cervix and the cervical canal even allowing visualization of preovulatory mucus; localization and delineation of uterine myomata and malformations and structures in the parametrium, visualization of gestational sacs and the site of implantation, early detection of multiple pregnancies after multiple embryo replacement, visualization of amnion, chorion, and fetal tissues, and guidance for chorionic biopsy procedures (3). A missing IUCD can be located, the fallopian tube entering the uterine cavity can be visualized and hydrosalpinges and abnormal pregnancy states can be picked up. Cancer of the ovary and endometrium can be screened.

2. In Obstetrics

Sexing of the baby can be obtained as early as 16 weeks and placenta praevia seen more clearly than through an abdominal scan. Determination of the cervical dilatation in cases of premature labour can be easily made as is accurate pelvimetry. Recently, a new transvaginal Doppler equipment has been developed and when combined with the transvaginal probe it allows pelvic blood flow measurements (ovarian and uterine arteries, umbilical cord, fetal aorta, etc) to be made (6).

REFERENCES

1. Lenz S, Lauritsen J G. Ultrasonically guided percutaneous aspiration of human follicles under local anesthesia: A new method of collecting oocytes for in vitro fertilization. Fertil. Steril. 1982; 38:673
2. Wilkand M, Nilsson L, Hansson R, Hamberger L, Janson P O. Collection of human oocytes by the use of sonography. Fertil. Steril. 1983; 39:603
3. Feichtinger W, Kemeter P. Tranvaginal sector scan sonography for needle-guided transvaginal follicle aspiration and other applications in gynecologic routine and research. Fertil. Steril. 1986; 42:722
4. Kemeter P, Feichtinger W. Transvaginal oocyte retrieval using a transvaginal sector scan probe combined with an automated puncture device. Hum. Reprod. 1986; 1:21
5. Feichtinger W, Kemeter P. Ultrasonically guided follicle aspiration as the method of choice for oocyte recovery for in vitro fertilization. In: Proceedings of the Fourth World Congress on IVF, Melbourne, Pelnum Press, New York, (in press)
6. Feichtinger W, Kemeter P, Putz M. New aspects of vaginal ultrasound in an IVF program Presented at the Fifth World Congress in IVF, Norfolk, proceedings published by The New York Academy of Sciences, in press.

9

Prostaglandins and Fertility Regulation

MARC BYGDEMAN

INTRODUCTION

A medical method for termination of early pregnancy would be an attractive alternative to vacuum aspiration, especially if the treatment could be administered by the woman herself. A prerequisite for such a procedure is that the treatment results in a complete abortion. Some of the naturally occurring prostaglandins (PGs), PGE_2 and PGF_{2alpha}, as well as certain analogues have the unique capacity to effectively stimulate uterine contractility during all stages of pregnancy. If the treatment is applied during the 4th to 7th week of pregnancy experience indicates that it is possible to achieve a high proportion of complete abortion. As the pregnancy advances the frequency of incomplete abortion increases and a medical method becomes less useful (1).

In the initial trials PGE_2 and PGF_{2alpha} were used (2). Although the treatment was able to terminate early pregnancy a high frequency of gastrointestinal side effects limited the clinical usefulness of the therapy (3). It was found that gastrointestinal side effects were reduced if the compounds were administered directly into the uterine cavity (4). However, this route of administration has obvious practical drawbacks limiting its clinical usefulness.

TERMINATION OF EARLY PREGNANCY BY PROSTAGLANDIN ANALOGUES

During recent years PGE_2 and PGF_{2alpha} have been replaced in clinical practice by prostaglandin analogues, eg 16,16-dimethyl-transΔ^2-PGE_1 (Cervagem; May & Baker, England), 16-phenoxy-tetranor-PGE_2 methyl sulfonylamide (Nalodor; Schering AG, Berlin) and 9-deoxo-16,16-dimethyl-9-methylene PGE_2 (9-methylene PGE_2; Upjohn Co, Kalamazoo) for preoperative dilatation of the cervical canal and for second trimester abortions. Treatment with these compounds is associated with a significantly lower frequency of side effects and can be administered either vaginally (9-methylene PGE_2 and Cervagem) or by the intramuscular route (Nalodor) (5).

The efficacy and safety of these three PGE analogues for termination of early pregnancy has been evaluated in a number of studies (6-10). In one of these studies the three PGE analogues were compared (8). The study involved almost 200 patients in early pregnancy (up to 49 days of amenorrhea) treated with either 0.5 mg 16-phenoxy PGE_2 three times with three hours interval, 0.5 mg Cervagem five times with the same time interval, of 75 and 30 mg or 60 and 45 mg with six hours interval. All three types of treatment were found equally effective resulting in complete abortion in 92 - 94% of the patients. Approximately 50% of the patients experienced occasional gastrointestinal side effects. Strong uterine pain necessitating analgesic treatment occurred in between 35% (for the E analogues administered by the vaginal route) and 56% (for Nalodor) of cases. In another study, one group of patients were allowed to treat themselves at home (11). The compound used was 9-methylene PGE_2 administered vaginally. Treatment of the patients was found to be equally effective in both those who had therapy at home as well as those in the hospital who were managed by research nurses. Only four patients had to return to hospital during the treatment because of strong uterine pain. None of the patients terminated the treatment because of side effects. The clinical events following treatment were very similar following either vaginal or intramuscular administration. All analogues induced an increase in uterine contractility followed by vaginal bleeding which generally started 3 to 6 hours after initiation of therapy and lasted 1 to 2 weeks. The total blood loss during non-surgical abortion in early pregnancy following treatment with different PG analogues varied between a mean of 61 and 131 ml (8, 12).

COMPARISON WITH VACUUM ASPIRATION

In a number of studies prostaglandin treatment and vacuum aspiration were randomly compared. All these studies showed that administration of PGF_2 directly into the uterine cavity (13) or vaginal or intramuscular administration of PGE analogues were as effective as vacuum aspiration for termination of early pregnancy (14-17). However, vacuum aspiration required less hospital time, caused fewer gastrointestinal side effects and resulted in a shorter period of bleeding and less blood loss. The WHO study (17) comprised a large number of patients (n = 474) in early pregnancy with amenorrhea of 49 days or less. The patients were randomly allocated to either three intramuscular injections of 0.5 mg Nalodor given at three hours interval or vacuum aspiration. Since a positive pregnancy test was not a prerequisite for entering the study the outcome of both procedures in non-pregnant women with a delay of menstruation due to reasons other than pregnancy could also be evaluated. The treatment was regarded as successful if the patients were not pregnant at the second follow-up visit two weeks after therapy, and curettage was not performed during the time period up to the first menstruation. Both the surgical and the non-surgical treatments were found equally effective, successful in 92.1% and 94.7% of cases respectively. The patients treated with the PGE analogue experienced gastrointestinal side effects and uterine pain more commonly than those undergoing vacuum aspiration. The duration of bleeding was also longer and the amount of blood loss heavier than the patients' own menstrual bleeding. The patients who were pregnant also started to bleed following PG therapy but the duration of bleeding and amount of blood loss was less. None of the patients experienced heavy bleeding and post-treatment infection was found to be equally rare following both treatments.

In another study the acceptability of prostaglandin treatment was evaluated (16). Vaginal administration of 9-methylene PGE_2 at home or in the hospital was randomly compared with vacuum aspiration. The study included 53 patients in early pregnancy (up to 49 days of amenorrhea) equally distributed between the three treatment groups. The patients were interviewed by a psychologist before and two weeks after treatment. Both the surgical and the non-surgical procedures were positively received. A majority of the patients treated with prostaglandins intended to use the same procedure in the event of a repeat abortion being required and would also recommend the treatment to a relative or friend. The results of this study indicate that termination of early pregnancy by a medical method, even if self-administered, is today an acceptable method in selected patients.

COMBINATION OF ANTIPROGESTIN AND PROSTAGLANDIN

As described previously, treatment with PGE analogues is equally effective as vacuum aspiration in terminating early pregnancy but side effects in terms of vomiting, diarrhoea and uterine pain limit the clinical use of this non-surgical procedure. Preliminary clinical data indicate that these problems can be substantially reduced if combined therapy using an antiprogestin and a prostaglandin is used. RU 486 is a steroid with a chemical structure similar to progesterone developed by the pharmaceutical company Roussel Uclaf (Paris, France). This compound competes with progesterone at the receptor sites and is believed to act mainly locally in the uterus causing decidual necrosis and detachment of the conceptus (18). The results of several clinical studies indicate that oral administration of RU 486 to early pregnant women in almost all cases induced vaginal bleeding but that the frequency of complete abortion, between 60 and 85%, was too low to compete with vacuum aspiration (19-23). Another problem was excessive bleeding which occurred in approximately 5% of the patients; gastrointestinal side effects and uterine pain rarely caused any problems for the patients (19, 20).

Normally, the early pregnant uterus is an inactive organ and no uterine contractions can be recorded. If a low dose of RU 486, 25 mg twice daily, is administered for 36 hours or more the treatment will result in the appearance of regular uterine contractions possibly by releasing the myometrium from the inhibitory effect of progesterone. As a result of the treatment the sensitivity of the myometrium to the stimulatory action of prostaglandin is also enhanced (23). In a recent clinical study a group of women in early pregnancy who were admitted for therapeutic abortion received 25 or 50 mg RU 486 twice daily for four days and a small dose of the PGE analogue (Nalodor, 0.25 mg i.m. or 1/4 to 1/6 of the dose needed if this analogue is used alone) was given in the morning of the fourth day. This type of combination therapy might be regarded as more physiological than giving each compound alone. There are reasons to believe that the increase in uterine contractility which occurs during a spontaneous abortion is preceded by a decrease in the influence of progesterone locally and an increase of endogenous PG biosynthesis.

The outcome of the study, which included 74 patients in early pregnancy, was promising. 96% of the patients aborted completely, no gastrointestinal side effects or heavy bleeding was recorded, and only eight patients experienced painful uterine contractions shortly after the prostaglandin treatment necessitating analgesic therapy. This first attempt to use a combination of an antiprogestin and a prostaglandin thus indicates that the procedure can be developed into a highly effective non-surgical method with fewer side effects than if PG analogues are used alone. Naturally, further studies are needed to prove the high efficacy of the method and to find out the most suitable treatment schedule. Preferably, the PG analogue should be administered orally as RU 486 to allow the patient to administer the treatment herself.

CONCLUSIONS

The present short review shows that the three PG analogues, Cervagem, Nalodor and 9-methylene PGE_2 are highly effective in terminating early pregnancy. The frequency of complete abortion is the same as for vacuum aspiration. However, the duration of bleeding is longer and frequency of uterine pain and gastrointestinal side effects is higher. In spite of these side effects the non-surgical procedure is often preferred by a majority of the patients treated with PGs, especially if self-administered. Treatment with the antiprogestin, RU 486, results in uterine bleeding in almost all patients but the frequency of complete abortion is unsatisfactory. If a low dose of a PGE analogue is added the rate of complete abortion increases significantly. The frequency of side effects is lower than if PGE analogues are used alone. It is realistic to believe that a combined treatment of an antiprogestin and a PG analogue will be developed into a competitive self-administered non-surgical alternative to vacuum aspiration for termination of early pregnancy.

ACKNOWLEDGEMENTS

Most studies referred to in this review and performed in our department were supported by WHO Special Programme on Research, Development and Research Training in Human Reproduction, Geneva, Switzerland. I am also grateful to Astrid Haggblad for skilful typing of the manuscript.

REFERENCES

1. Bygdeman M, Borell U, Leader A, Lundstrom V, Martin JN Jr, Eneroth P, Green K. Induction of first and second trimester abortion by the vaginal administration of 15-methyl PGF$_{2alpha}$ methyl ester. In: Samuelsson B, and Paoletti R (Eds) Advances in Prostaglandin and Thromboxane Research, Vol 2 Raven Press, New York 1976, pp 693-704

2. Karim SMM. Once a month vaginal administration of prostaglandin E$_2$ and F$_2$ for fertility control. Contraception 1971; 3:173-183

3. Tredway DR, Mishell DR. Therapeutic abortion of early human gestation with vaginal suppositories of prostaglandin F$_{2alpha}$. Am J Obstet Gynecol 1973; 116:795-798

4. Csapo AI, Kivikoski A, Wiest WG. Massive initial prostaglandin impact in postconceptional therapy. Prostaglandins 1972; 2:125-134

5. Lauersen NH. Induced abortion. In: Bygdeman M, Berger GS and Keith LG (Eds) Prostaglandins and their Inhibitors in Clinical Obstetrics and Gynecology. MTP Press Ltd, Lancaster 1986, pp 271-314

6. Karim SMM, Rao B, Ratnam SS, Prasad RNV, Wong YM, Ilancheran A. Termination of early pregnancy (menstrual induction) with 16-phenoxy-w-tetranor-PGE$_2$ methyl sulfonylamide. Contraception 1977; 16:377-381

7. Fleischer A, Schulman H, Blattner P, Jagani N, Fayemi A. Early pregnancy-abortion model using sulprostone. Prostaglandins 1982; 23:643-655

8. Bygdeman M, Christensen NJ, Green K, Zheng S, Lundstrom V. Termination of early pregnancy - future development. Acta Obstet Gynecol Scand Suppl 1983; 113:125-129

9. Karim SMM, Ratnam SS, Ilancheran A Menstrual induction with vaginal administration of 16,16-dimethyl-trans-Δ-PGE$_1$ methyl ester (ONO-802). Prostaglandins 1977; 14:615-616

10. WHO Prostaglandin Task Force. Termination of early first trimester pregnancy by vaginal administration of 16,16-dimethyl-trans-Δ-PGE$_1$ methyl ester. Asia Oceania J Obstet Gynecol 1982; 8:263-268

11. Bygdeman M, Christensen NJ, Green K and Vesterqvist O. Self-administration at home of prostaglandin for termination of early pregnancy. In: Toppozada M, Bygdeman M and Hafez ESE (Eds) Prostaglandins and Fertility Regulation, MTP Press Ltd, Lancaster, 1984 pp 83-90

12. Hamberger L, Nilsson B, Bjorn-Rasmussen E, Atterfelt P, Wiqvist N. Early abortion by vaginal prostaglandin suppositories. Contraception 1977; 17:183-194

13. Ragab MJ, Edelman D. Early termination of pregnancy. A comparative study of cintrauterine PGF$_2$ and vacuum aspiration. Prostaglandins 1976; 11:275-283

14. Lundstrom V, Bygdeman M, Fotiou S, Green K, Kinoshita K. Abortion in early pregnancy by vaginal administration of 16,16-dimethyl-PGE$_2$ in comparison with vacuum aspiration. Contraception 1977; 16:167-173

15. Rosen AS, Nystedt I, Bygdeman M, Lundstrom V. Acceptability of a non-surgical method to terminate very early pregnancy in comparison to vacuum aspiration. Contraception 1979; 19:107-117

16. Rosen AS, von Knorring K, Bygdeman M, Christensen N. Randomized comparison of prostaglandin treatment in hospital or at home with vacuum aspiration for termination of early pregnancy. Contraception 1984; 29:423-435

17. WHO Task Force on Postovulatory Methods for Fertility Control Menstrual regulation by intramuscular injection of 16-phenoxy-tetranor PGE_2 methyl sulfonylamide. Br J Obstet Gynaecol 1987 (in press).
18. Baulieu EE. An antiprogestin steroid with contragestive activity in women. In: Baulieu EE and Segal SJ (Eds) The Antiprogestin Steroid RU 486 and Human Fertility Control. Plenum Press, New York, 1985 pp 1-26
19. Herrman W, Wyss R, Riondel A. The effects of an anti-progesterone steroid in women; Interruption of the menstrual cycle and of early pregnancy. Comptes Rendus 1982; 294:933-938
20. Kovacs L, Sas M, Resch B. Termination of very early pregnancy by RU 486, an antiprogestational compound. Contraception 1984; 29:399-409
21. Sitruk-Ware R, Billaued L, Mowszowica I. The use of RU 486 as an abortifacient in early pregnancy. In: Baulieu EE and Segal SJ (Eds) The Antiprogestin Steroid RU 486 and Human Fertility Control. Plenum Press, New York, 1985 pp 243-248
22. Schaison G. Contragestion with mifepristone. In: Diczfalusy E and Bygdeman M (Eds) Fertility Regulation Today and Tomorrow. Serono Symposia Publications, Vol 36, Raven Press, New York, 1987 pp 105-108
23. Bygdeman M, Swahn ML. Progesterone receptor blockage. Effect on uterine contractility and early pregnancy. Contraception 1985; 32:45-51
24. Swahn ML, Bygdeman M Interruption of early gestation with prostaglandins and antiprogestin. In: Diczfalusy E and Bygdeman M (Eds) Fertility Regulation Today and Tomorrow. Serono Symposia Publications, Vol 36, Raven Press, New York, 1987 pp 109-118

Index